weights
FOR
women

**CREATE A BEAUTIFUL
BODY IN LESS THAN
AN HOUR A WEEK!**

Ian Endacott

D0532822

Dorset County Library		
Askews	2009	
613.71082	£9.99	

Dorset Libraries
Withdrawn Stock

DORSET COUNTY LIBRARY

204741134 Q

MW

An Hachette Livre UK Company
www.hachettelivre.co.uk

First published in Great Britain in 2009 by Hamlyn,
a division of Octopus Publishing Group Ltd
2–4 Heron Quays, London E14 4JP
www.octopusbooks.co.uk

Copyright © Octopus Publishing Group Ltd 2009

All rights reserved. No part of this work may
be reproduced or utilized in any form or by any
means, electronic or mechanical, including
photocopying, recording or by any information
storage and retrieval system, without the
prior written permission of the publisher.

Jan Endacott asserts the moral right to be
identified as the author of this work.

ISBN: 978-0-600-61637-5

A CIP catalogue record for this book is available
from the British Library.

Printed and bound in China.

10 9 8 7 6 5 4 3 2 1

All reasonable care has been taken in the
preparation of this book, but the information it
contains is not meant to take the place of medical
care under the direct supervision of a doctor.
Before making any changes in your health regime,
always consult a doctor. Any application of the
ideas and information contained in this book is at
the reader's sole discretion and risk. Neither the
author nor the publisher will be responsible for
any injury, loss, damages, actions, proceedings,
claims, demands, expenses and costs (including
legal costs or expenses) incurred in any way
arising out of following exercises in this book.

**Jan Endacott trained for 12 years at the
acclaimed Bush Davies Ballet School and
subsequently travelled the world enjoying a
successful career as a professional dancer and
dance teacher. She then qualified as a personal
fitness coach, sports psychologist and Pilates
instructor, specializing in women's fitness. Her
exercise programmes have enabled women of all
ages and abilities to achieve their personal
fitness goals. Jan is also author of *The Fitball
Workout* and *Pilates for Pregnancy*.**

CONTENTS

INTRODUCTION

Working with weights will surprise you! You are about to discover the amazing advantages that weight training will bring to your life. If you are wondering how to get started, this book will help you to decide what equipment you need and to weight train safely and effectively. The easy-to-follow format will guide you comfortably through your chosen programmes.

You don't need expensive or bulky equipment to follow the exercises, which can be done at home in your own time. Follow one of the workout programmes provided at the end of the book, each of which comprises a set of 10 exercises, perform this twice a week – and in less than an hour per week you will be on your way to achieving your goals!

How to use this book

Read the rest of this chapter first. It will guide you through understanding how your muscles work, the importance of correct posture, starting safely and basic fitness tests. You will learn how to choose equipment and follow essential training guidelines, and how to motivate yourself to achieve the best possible results.

This is followed by chapters on Warm-up and Cool-Down Stretches, and exercises for the Upper Body, Mid-Section Body and Lower Body. Read the information provided at the start of each chapter and then study the exercises that follow. Then choose an appropriate workout from the menus on pages 116–125: there are programmes to suit everyone. Stick with your chosen workout for at least four weeks and you will be delighted with the results. Happy exercising!

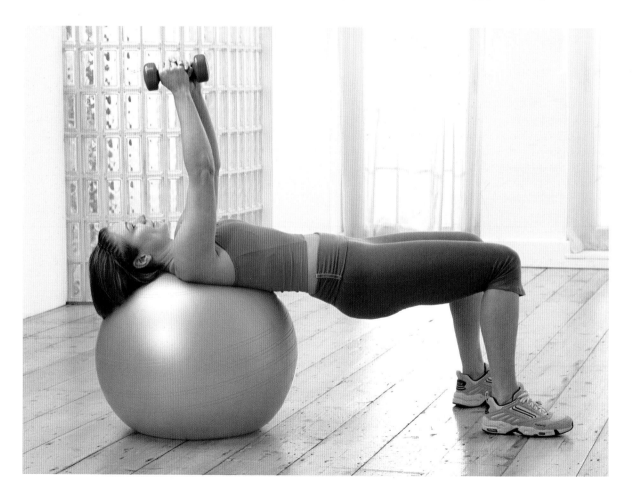

why use weights?

Weight training provides superb exercise, and more and more women are using weights to enhance their feminine curves. Apart from the cosmetic benefits, there are real health advantages to using weights. The workouts in this book will help you look and feel younger, stronger, more energetic, and boost your self-confidence. These benefits are too good to ignore.

Helps to reduce body fat Weight training replaces fat with muscle. With more lean muscle you will look slimmer and more compact. The more lean muscle you acquire, the better. Lean muscle helps you to burn up calories and fat long after you have finished exercising, because your metabolism remains raised for longer.

Improves bone density Osteoporosis is a silent disease that sabotages our bones, making them brittle and porous due to loss of bone density. It affects one in three women over the age of 50. Performing regular strength training twice weekly helps to improve and preserve bone density, even in post-menopausal women. Improved strength and balance also reduces the risk of falls, which are a common cause of fractures in those suffering from osteoporosis.

Reduces blood pressure Weight training has been shown to reduce resting blood pressure. Heart disease and strokes are still the most common cause of death and carrying excess weight increases this risk. Regular physical activity (coupled with a healthy diet) is of huge benefit. A stronger body means less strain on the heart, and structured strength training – alongside regular cardiovascular (aerobic) exercise for the heart and lungs – will help to reduce hypertension.

Alleviates arthritis and joint pain Millions of people suffer from various diseases of the joints. Being overweight exacerbates this as the hips, knees and ankles bear the full weight load. Maintaining strong muscles is essential for sufferers, yet many shy away as they fear more discomfort or risk of further damage to the joints. Moderate weight training will help to ease pain and increase mobility in joints, while strong muscles help to support the bones.

Reduces the risk of diabetes This disease is sweeping western society and contributing to heart disease. Regular weight training appears to improve glucose metabolism (poor glucose metabolism is

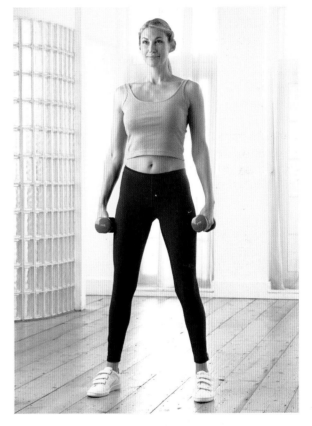

linked to the onset of diabetes in adults). More exercise will also reduce obesity, which itself is linked to diabetes.

Improves self-confidence and self-esteem Regular weight training boosts your self-image, making you feel more confident and empowered. It can help to alleviate depression as endorphins – hormones released when you exercise – surge, making you feel happy.

Helps you to stay young Stress, fatigue and muscle loss are ageing. Weight training can reduce stress levels and help you to sleep better. By gaining more muscle you will look great and burn more fat. What better reason do you need to make a start right now?

understanding your muscles

The human body is beautifully designed but needs regular activity to maintain peak physical condition. Without use, muscle tone will deteriorate, causing muscular imbalances, pain and eventually even debilitating disease. Few of us achieve even a small proportion of the level of activity that, combined with a balanced diet, is necessary for overall good health.

Understanding what your muscles do is the first step towards successful training, helping you to apply your thought process for superb targeted results. Your body has nearly 700 muscles. Some work involuntarily without conscious control, like your heart. The voluntary (skeletal) muscles attach to your bones by ligaments and tendons. If you do not work these voluntary muscles they will become weak, affecting your ability to perform simple activities such as walking, lifting and carrying. Long-term inactivity will also weaken involuntary muscles, like the heart. The result will be loss of strength, balance, endurance and stamina, eventually resulting in serious illness.

It is not necessary to be an expert on muscular anatomy and you may well ask, "do I really need to know about all this?". The answer is yes. A simple understanding of where your muscles are positioned and the way they respond to exercise, will help you progress more effectively and gain the best results.

The muscle groups that improve your appearance and enhance your overall shape are the chest, back, shoulders, bicep, tricep, gluteals, hamstrings, quadriceps, calves and abdominals. These major muscle groups consist of individual muscles, which generally act as secondary movers in a stabilizing role. The charts opposite (page 7) show the location of each muscle group, and it is these main muscles that have the most influence on your overall shape and appearance.

Knowing where muscles are located enables you to focus your thoughts and concentrate mentally on the area of the body you are exercising. For example, when you are performing an exercise that targets the gluteal (buttock) muscles, you should think about really squeezing the buttock muscles strongly whilst imagining the firm, pert rounded bottom that is your goal. This technique is called visualization, and is widely used to enable sportspeople to improve performance.

Such mental awareness creates a mind-to-muscle pathway that encourages a fine-tuned response from the working muscles. In turn, this improves your exercise technique through strong, correct movement quality, better control of your weights, and results in good body alignment.

This heightened self-awareness will help you to gain the very best from your body that will show in better posture, more strength, and the achievement of the image and shape you have set as your goals. The bonus is improved self-confidence and self-esteem, which will help you to naturally develop a positive attitude to life!

Working with weights will help to maintain a healthy, balanced body free from the constant pain associated with imbalances, postural problems, joint pain and preventable diseases such as osteoporosis (see page 5). Act now to promote your future health and vitality.

Front view

Back view

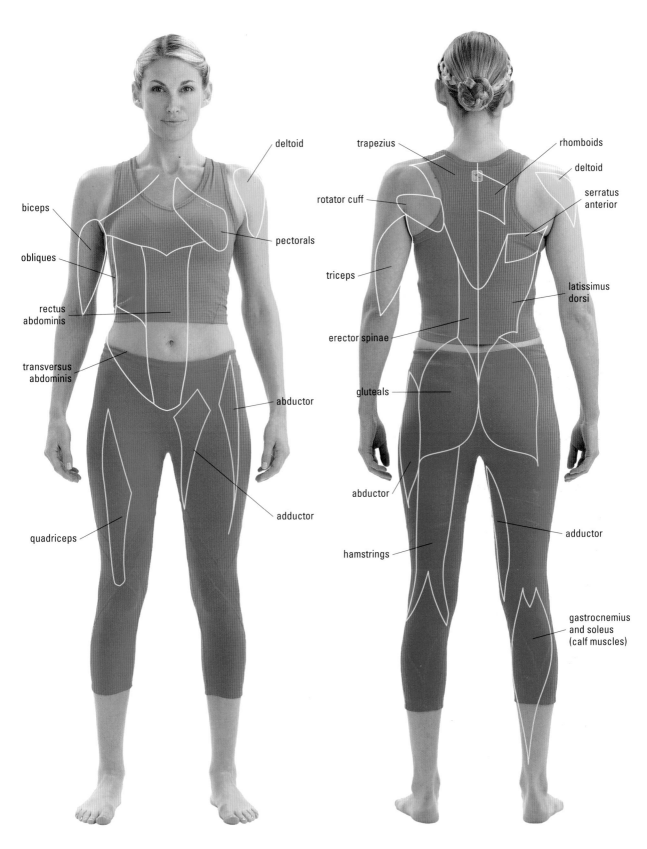

- deltoid
- biceps
- obliques
- pectorals
- rectus abdominis
- transversus abdominis
- abductor
- adductor
- quadriceps
- trapezius
- rhomboids
- deltoid
- rotator cuff
- serratus anterior
- triceps
- latissimus dorsi
- erector spinae
- gluteals
- abductor
- adductor
- hamstrings
- gastrocnemius and soleus (calf muscles)

posture and balance

Correct posture is vital to good health, influencing your long-term general wellbeing. Standing with good alignment will reduce the stress on your back and joints. Well-trained, balanced muscles provide a support structure for your bone framework. A little time spent laying the foundations of good posture will provide fantastic benefits.

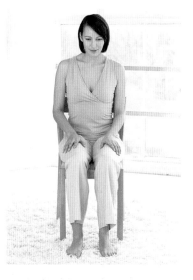

Core connector

The deep-seated muscles of your stomach and back provide stability for your spine. To improve posture and flatten your stomach, practise the following exercise daily.

1 Sit comfortably on a chair or cross-legged on the mat, and place your fingertips 5 cm (2 in) in and 5 cm (2 in) down from your hipbones.

2 To lift your pelvic floor, imagine sitting on a diamond shape. Breathe out, and draw the four corners of the diamond inward and upward, simultaneously pulling your navel towards your spine. Feel your muscles tighten. Hold for as long as is comfortable while breathing normally, then release. Perform 3–5 repetitions.

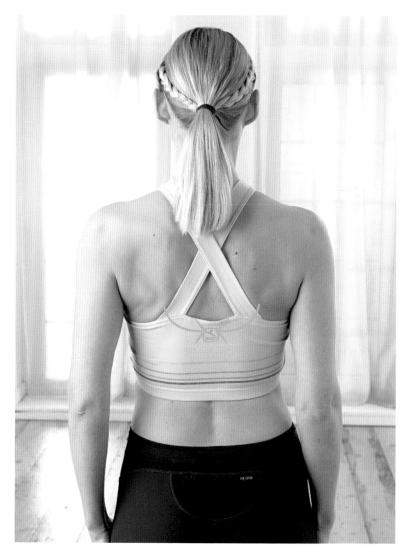

Anchor your shoulder blades

Anchoring your shoulder blades avoids upper body imbalance and prevents rounded shoulders, which are ageing and very unattractive! Try this simple movement to correct your posture.

Draw your shoulder blades down and slightly inwards. Practise this 'anchoring' routine daily to help you develop good upper body posture and stand with poise.

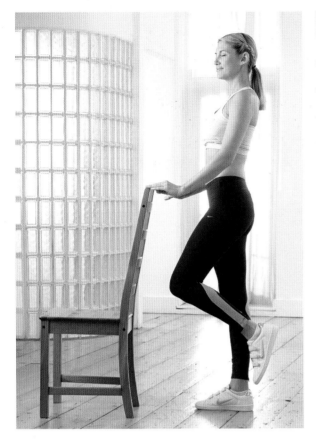
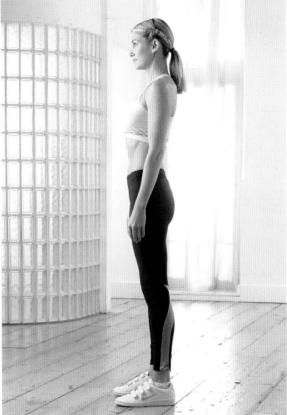

Balance

Accidental falls often occur in later life and may cause serious injury to those with osteoporosis. Strength training improves balance and co-ordination, while exercising on the stability ball enhances balance and core stability by providing an unstable surface. (For more information on the ball see page 14; for how to get on and off it safely, see pages 78 and 82.) Practise this simple exercise every day to improve your balance.

Place a sturdy chair beside you for support if you need it. Keeping your eyes closed, lift one foot from the floor and hold for 15–20 seconds. Repeat on the opposite side.

Standing tall

Standing tall with good alignment will ensure that you maintain essential good posture.

1 Stand sideways-on to a full-length mirror, with your feet positioned under your hipbones. Think of each foot as a triangle, distributing your weight evenly through the heel, the ball of the big toe and your little toe. Pull up through the arches of your feet.

2 Keep your knees relaxed, not overly bent or locked. Keep your hips square and level.

3 Check in the mirror that your pelvis is not tilted forward or back. Neutral spine alignment is halfway between a full tilt forward and back, with the lower back following a slight, natural curve inwards.

4 Lengthen through your spine. Gently draw your navel towards your spine, with ribs stacked above hipbones.

5 Open and lift your chest. Gently slide your shoulder blades down and slightly into the back of your ribs.

6 Your head should be balanced freely on your neck, eyes looking straight ahead. Keep your chin level and pulled back slightly.

getting started

Before embarking on any new form of exercise, be completely honest with yourself. If you have any health concerns that may be aggravated by exercise, your progress will be impaired. Study the advice below to enable you to proceed safely and get the best from your training.

Before you start

Always consult your doctor before starting any exercise programme, especially if any of the following apply:

- Your chest hurts when you are physically active.
- You have a heart condition.
- You have felt any chest pain recently when you are not doing physical activity.
- You suffer from loss of balance or dizzy spells, or are prone to fainting.
- You suffer from high blood pressure.
- You have problems with your muscles, bones or joints that worsen when you are active.
- You are pregnant.

If you are not aware of any of the above, or any other reason you should not exercise, you can get started. However, it is essential to begin slowly and gradually so that your body can adapt to the demands placed on it. Don't overdo it!

Keeping it going

Following these simple rules will ensure that you make steady progress in your training and avoid unnecessary setbacks:

Warm-up Always begin your weights workout with a 5-minute warm-up. This activates your muscles and provides you with time to mentally prepare. Never skip the after-training stretches (the cool-down), which restore the muscles to their natural resting length and increase flexibility. Warm-up and cool-down stretches are covered on pages 22–39.

Breathe Remember to breathe. It is very common for people new to exercise to hold their breath. A general rule is to breathe out on the effort and in on the release. If in doubt, breathe naturally.

Pain Pain means your body is telling you to STOP! It indicates that something is wrong, and working through pain may cause you serious damage.

Illness Avoid exercise when you are ill. Your immune system is fighting back, and you need your reserves to help your body repair itself.

Exercise environment

Make sure you have enough room and a clear floor space. Keep the room temperature even: too hot and you will be uncomfortable, too cold and your muscles will be tense. Wear suitable, comfortable clothes that allow freedom of movement.

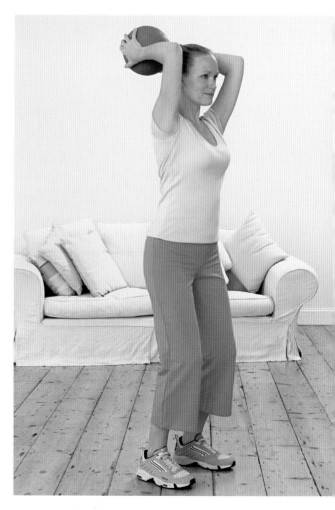

Drinking and eating

Ensure you consume enough fluid before, during and after exercise. If you feel thirsty, you are already dehydrated. Water plays a vital role in regulating body temperature and you need to drink at least eight glasses a day – more when exercising and in raised temperatures. Drink small amounts often. Try not to eat during the two hours prior to exercising.

Cardiovascular exercise

For complete fitness, include daily cardiovascular exercise in addition to your weight training programme to keep your heart and lungs healthy.

Walking is a great choice as it's easy to do anywhere. Aim for 30 minutes a day, less if you're unfit, or break it down into 10-minute chunks throughout the day. Build up the time gradually as you adapt to your weight training, otherwise the first few weeks will be too tiring. Walk with a purpose (imagine you are late for an important appointment), swinging your arms in a pumping action and pushing off from your back foot.

Swimming and cycling are non-impact exercises that are easy on the joints. For the energetic, aerobics, skipping, hula-hooping or dancing will increase your heart rate.

Know your body type

Recognizing your genetic body type will help you to achieve your end goals. Most of us are made up of two categories, for example ectomorph/mesomorph (see below). Having a totally honest picture of how you look now and what is realistically possible (10 cm/4 in extra leg length is not!) will help you to fulfil your expectations.

There are three basic body types:

Endomorph Narrow shoulders, short limbs, long torso and wide hips with a soft, rounded shape. Choose exercises to balance your shape. Increase your upper body size, strength and shoulder width using heavier weights. Perform a high number of repetitions with light weights for your lower body.

Ectomorph Short upper torso, long limbs, narrow chest and shoulders. Lean with little fat, ectomorphs have difficulty gaining muscle. Consistent weight training provides best results. Pay particular attention to posture and protect your joints, which will help you to guard against osteoporosis.

Mesomorph Muscular, athletic body, broad shoulders, large chest, ribcage well developed to the waist, powerful calves and forearms. Mesomorphs are strong and gain muscle easily so must balance their workouts carefully, aiming for shape not bulk. Go for variety, performing exercises that use your own body weight, and do plenty of cardiovascular work.

analyzing your fitness

Having followed the safety checks and you are sure you have no other health concerns (see pages 10–11), you are ready to begin. The following basic fitness tests are simple and will provide a starting point, allowing you to monitor your progress during the coming months. For subsequent tests (each time you move on to a new workout programme, or after six to eight weeks' training) perform the same Press-ups and Ab-Curls so that the results are reproduceable. Warm up for about 5 minutes before doing either of the muscular fitness tests, using movements from pages 25–30.

Press-up test

Test your upper body strength by seeing how many Half Press-ups you can do in 1 minute. (To establish correct technique, see page 44.) Count as many as you can perform with good quality.

- **Above average** 40 or more without rest
- **Average** 24–39
- **Below average** 23 or less

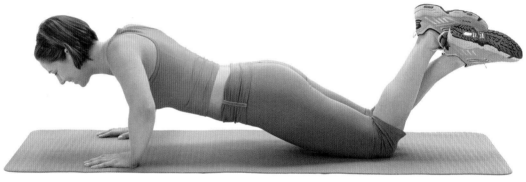

Ab-Curl test

Test your stomach muscle strength by seeing how many Ab-Curls you can do in 1 minute. (To establish correct technique, see page 76.) Count as many as you can perform with good technique.

- **Above average**
  45 or more
- **Average** 24–45
- **Below average**
  23 or less

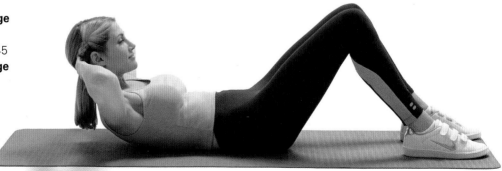

'Before' and 'after' photographs

Taking photos of yourself is possibly the greatest test of all, especially if you are unhappy with your body image. If you can muster up the courage, it really is a useful visual reminder of what you want to change. A 'before' photo of yourself in a swimsuit or underwear shows you exactly where you are now and what you want to improve. Keep to your training programme. You will then enjoy the satisfaction of seeing the discipline and hard work you've applied to your workouts paying off in positive results, with a new you looking back at you from the 'after' photos!

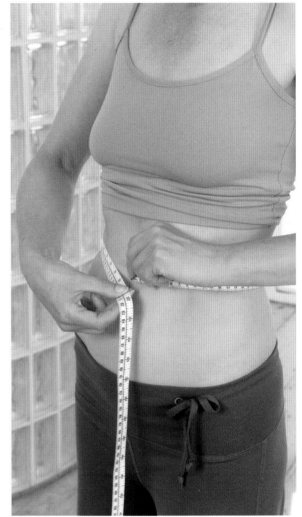

Hip-to-waist ratio

This test provides a good indication of your fat distribution and highlights potential health problems, since storing fat around your middle puts you at greater risk of obesity-linked disease. Measure your waist directly over your navel, then measure over the widest part of your hips. Divide your waist measurement by your hip measurement (use metric or imperial).

- **Above average** below 0.70
- **Average** 0.71–0.84
- **Below average** over 0.85

Flexibility

This movement tests flexibility in your spine and legs. Sit on the floor with your back against the wall, with your legs together and in front of you. Slowly reaching your fingertips forward, see how far down your legs you can reach without forcing or straining your back.

- **Above average** To shins or further
- **Average** To knees
- **Below average** Above knees

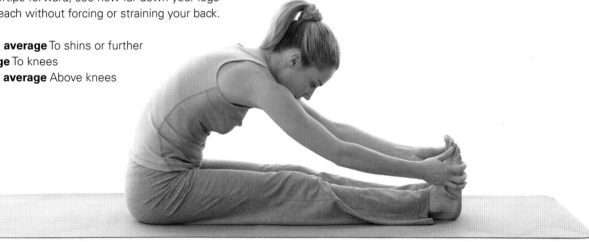

choosing equipment

With a huge range of home exercise equipment available, choose items that are versatile, durable and uncomplicated. The equipment needed for the exercises in this book is easy to use and inexpensive, allowing you to try out many exercise combinations. Variety helps maintain your interest and motivation, providing you with a great workout and effective progression.

Medicine ball

A good alternative to dumbbells, a weighted ball offers variety and provides an alternative training stimulus, which will enhance your progress and prevent boredom. Medicine balls are available in a range of weight increments: select a 2 kg (4½ lb) ball to start with, which will offer you medium resistance, and move on to a 3 kg (6½ lb) ball when you need more challenge.

Stability ball

Used as an alternative to a bench, a stability ball challenges your core muscles and can increase the intensity of exercises. It also improves your balance and co-ordination, so it really is a versatile and indispensable piece of equipment.

You will need to determine the correct ball size for you. The box below will help you select the appropriate ball size for your height and weight.

Choosing the correct ball size

When seated on the ball, your knees should be level with or slightly below your hips and bent at 90 degrees. Your feet should be flat on the floor. Your height is not the only determining factor: your weight is also relevant. For overweight, unfit or mature people, a larger ball that is slightly under-inflated is preferable. It is also easier to practise new or challenging exercises with the ball slightly under-inflated. A smaller, firmer ball will be more challenging to balance on than a larger, softer one. To inflate the ball, use a special ball pump or a foot pump with an appropriate adaptor.

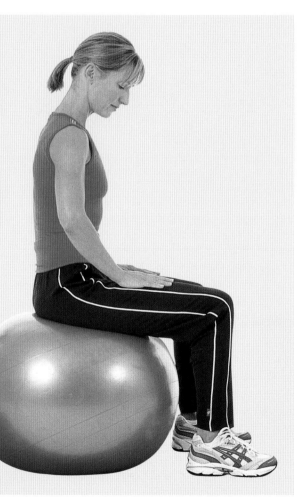

HEIGHT	BALL SIZE
under 1.57 m (5ft 2in)	45 cm (18 in)
1.60–1.73 m (5 ft 3 in–5 ft 8 in)	55 cm (22 in)
1.75–1.90 m (5 ft 9 in–6 ft 3 in)	65 cm (26 in)
1.93–2.06 m (6 ft 4 in–6 ft 9 in)	75 cm (30 in)

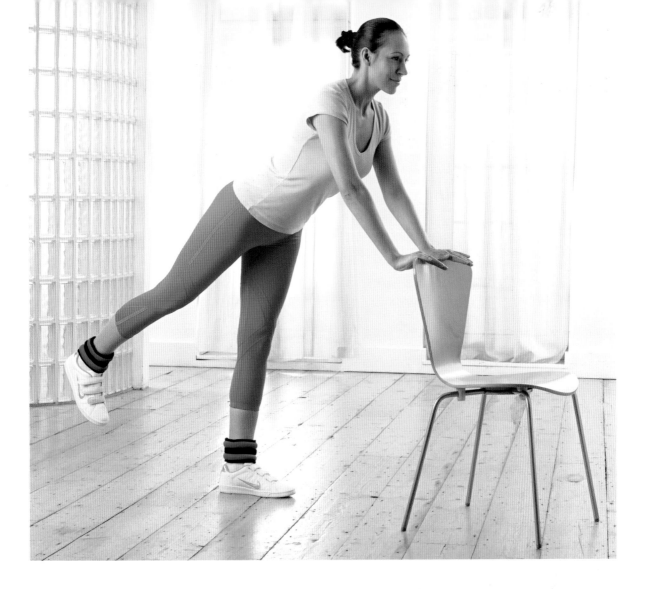

Ankle weights

These are soft, weighted cuffs with adjustable touch-and-close straps that attach around the ankle and provide weighted resistance for lower body training. Start with a pair of 1 kg (2¼ lb) cuffs, and when these are no longer challenging move on to 2 kg (4½ lb). Soft, seamless cuffs are the best choice and sit neatly in place. They can also be worn on the wrists if you have arthritis in your hands and find that holding dumbbells is difficult.

Dumbbells

Dumbbells are available in a range of materials, from chrome (some with rubber inlay) to steel dipped in vinyl or coated with neoprene. Some lighter-weight dumbbells have a foam covering and touch-and-close straps to prevent accidental release.

Neoprene dumbbells are the nicest to hold, do not slip in hot hands and are chip resistant. They are available in a variety of colours and many different weight combinations.

Be aware of safety considerations whenever you are using dumbbells. Take care when you lift them from the floor, always hold them firmly and do not leave them lying around ready for you to trip over.

As a temporary substitute, you can use food cans for hand weights until you are ready to purchase your own dumbbells.

Exercise mat

There is a vast array of mats available, from foam folding/roll-up styles to yoga 'sticky' mats. The mats that offer most support and durability are made from softer foam, which cushions your back and is non-slip. A thick towel can serve as a temporary substitute until you are ready to purchase a purpose-made mat.

Other equipment

Other useful pieces of equipment used in this book include soft foam balls, towels to fold or roll, and small and large cushions.

training guidelines

The exercises in this book are grouped into balanced workouts, designed to shape and strengthen all the muscles in your body. Choosing the best individual exercises for you means understanding basic training principles. Study the following pages and progress at a level that is both challenging and achievable, to help you stay on track and fit into your busy lifestyle.

Dispelling the myths

Weight training will not produce bulky muscles. You will only achieve bulk with vast amounts of testosterone (in short supply for women) and by using heavy weights with specific exercises, coupled with a diet designed to increase muscle bulk. Women become slimmer and more shapely through weight training because fat is reduced and lean muscle appears.

Weight training is good for overweight, underweight, unfit or older women. Take it slowly, starting with the Essential Workout (see page 118) and then progressing at your own individual pace. Achieving your best look means keeping your body's proportions balanced. For example, a pear shape needs a toned lower body matched with extra upper body work to balance proportions and draw the eye away from heavy hips. If you are looking to lose weight, training must be combined with daily cardiovascular exercise to achieve balance and best results.

The training framework

Some exercises, called multiple-joint or compound exercises, train several muscle groups simultaneously, while single-joint exercises focus on isolating one particular area.

Training should ensure that large muscles are exercised before small muscles. This maximizes training efficiency, because the larger muscles are stabilized by the smaller ones and you therefore need to avoid fatiguing the smaller ones first.

The workout programmes in this book (see pages 116–125) are designed to give you progressive and balanced training.

Reps, sets and rest

These terms are defined as follows:

Repetition (rep) One complete cycle of an exercise from the start position, through the whole movement and back to the start position. Each exercise will specify the number of reps you should perform.

Set Total number of reps you should complete continuously without rest. In this book, 1–3 sets are specified most often.

If, for example, 'reps 12–15, Sets 1' is specified, this means performing the exercise continuously 12–15 times before taking a break and moving on to the next exercise. If the exercise states 'reps 12–15, sets 2', you will repeat the exercise sequence 12–15 times, rest for about 30 seconds, and repeat the sequence continuously another 12–15 times.

Your current level of fitness dictates your starting level. As a general guide, a complete beginner should perform 1 set. When this becomes easier – remember that the last few reps of an exercise must be challenging – add another set. When 2 sets becomes easy, move on to 3 sets. Remember to rest for about 30 seconds between sets.

Lifting and lowering When performing weight-lifting repetitions, you should lift for a count of 2–3 seconds and lower for a count of 4 seconds. It's essential to appreciate that the lowering phase of a movement is as important as the lifting phase in achieving exercise benefits. A good example is the Biceps Beautifier (see page 59). As you lift the weights into the curl-up movement, the resistance of the weight ensures that you lift with effort and control. On the lowering phase, the weights are pulled down by gravity and therefore the tendency is to allow them to 'drop' back to the start position. You must not let this happen. Lower the weights slowly as you count 4 seconds so that you, not gravity, control the lowering. In this way you will gain maximum benefit from the complete exercise movement.

When to exercise Choose a time that suits you and your lifestyle and stick to it! Exercising first thing in the morning is often best as it gets you off to a flying start for the day.

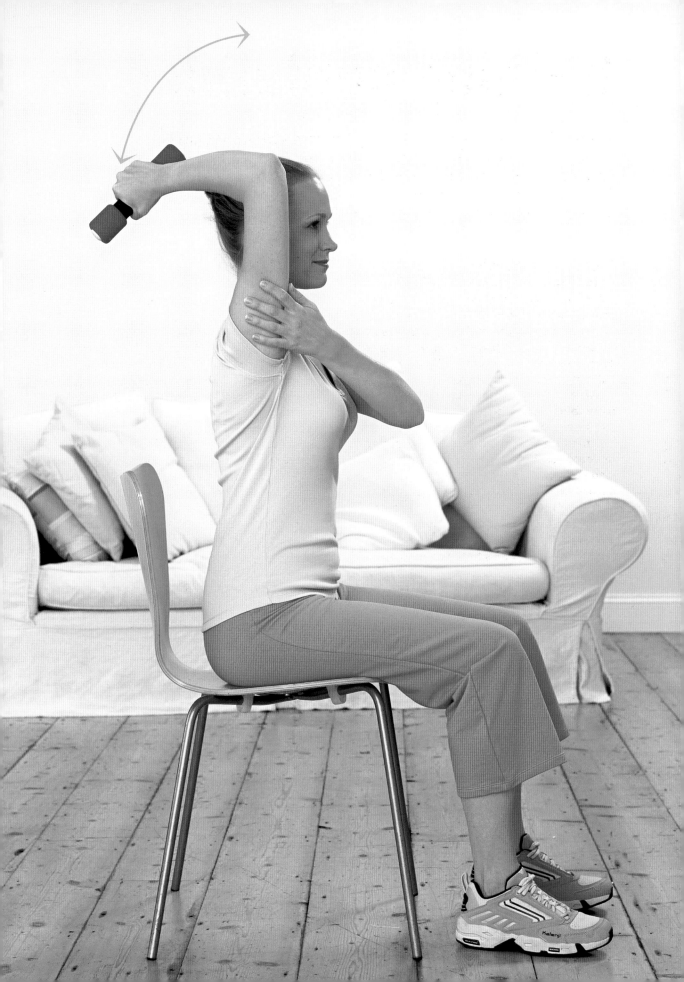

Weak and strong sides When performing exercises that work one side and then the other, always start with your weaker side to help balance your strength gains, as this side fatigues faster than the stronger side: if you exercise your weaker side second, overall fatigue may cause poor technique on this side due to lack of strength and therefore control. Exercising in the correct order also creates stronger nerve pathways and better balance.

Exercise order and frequency

To gain maximum benefit from your training, follow these guidelines:

■ Each workout should include 8–10 separate exercises that work all the major muscle groups (see pages 116–125).

■ Perform weight training twice a week in order to gain the desired results in the minimum time.
■ Ensure you take a rest period of at least 48 hours between workouts.
■ If you are pushed for time, split your workouts into four shorter sessions: for example, upper body on days 1 and 3, lower body on days 2 and 4.
■ Advanced exercisers may like to add a third session to their programme.
■ The amount of time it takes you to complete each workout depends largely on your familiarity with each movement and technique.
■ Whatever your starting point, progress gradually and be patient.
■ Consistency pays off, so stick with each workout for at least four weeks before moving on to a fresh programme.

Selecting weights

Ideally, you should purchase 3 pairs of dumbbells: light, medium and heavy. The medium-weight dumbbell is the one you can lift continuously 12 times when performing a Biceps Beautifier (see page 59). Then buy a pair of dumbbells 1 kg (2¼ 1b) lighter and a pair 1 kg (2¼ lb) heavier.

These three weights will accommodate all the dumbbell exercises and you will work out at the right level. The appropriate weight for each exercise will be the one you can lift continuously for the required number of reps, with the last 2 reps being an effort to complete. Once you can easily perform up to 15 reps with good form and little effort, it's time to increase the weight, so invest in dumbbells 1 kg (2¼ lb) heavier. This provides the extra stimulus (or 'progressive overload') for your body to continue to improve.

Techniques

Whenever possible, stand in front of a full-length mirror while performing each exercise. This will enable you to check your posture and quality of movement, helping you to assimilate and process these visual reminders quickly. Your muscle memory will then absorb these messages, creating more efficient patterns of movement each time you exercise. Consequently, each workout will become more effective as you hone and perfect your training technique, producing stronger, better results.

Always focus mentally on the muscles you are working (for example, imagine firm, rounded buttocks as you lift your leg behind you) to achieve enviable results. Engage your abdominal muscles continuously to protect your spine and perfect your technique.

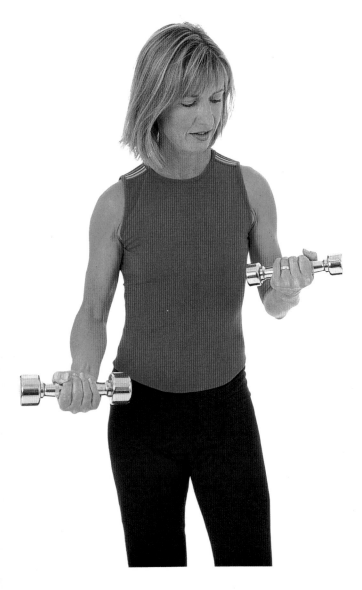

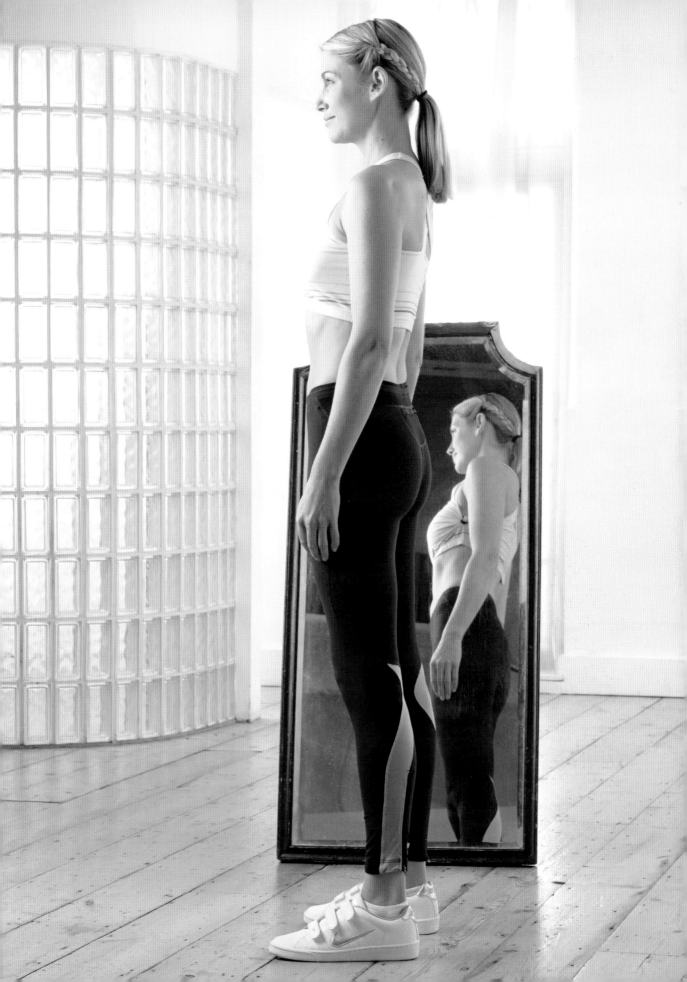

fitness with attitude

Achieve best results by establishing a positive mental attitude, banishing negative thoughts and developing a strategy of clearly defined goals. You need to plan specific steps towards your ultimate aim or it will remain just a dream. Identify exactly what you want and how you are going to get there. Make your goals real by writing them down in a fitness diary.

Believe in yourself

A strong unconscious drive exists in us all that compels us to behave consistently within our beliefs, which in turn affects our thoughts. Try changing the way you think about yourself: instead of seeing challenges as difficulties, see them as opportunities. Develop a positive attitude!

Setting goals

However busy you are, it is essential to pause long enough to think about what you really want and how you can achieve this. Your goals must be:

Balanced They should cater for all areas of your life. Devoting all your free time to exercising will overload you and could, for example, affect your relationships negatively, thereby actually hampering your progress. Great achievements need quality rest and inner calmness to help you focus.

Precise Write down a detailed description of what you really want and when you want it by. For example: 'Look fit in a new bikini for our holiday in eight weeks' time'.

Desirable They must be what you truly want.

Challenging Goals must push you to achieve your personal best.

Time-framed Set an 'achieve by' date to avoid drifting along aimlessly.

Long- and short-term goals

Identify your **long-term goals** first. For example, you may wish to take part in a charity power walk in 12 months' time. Writing down this long-term goal will make it a concrete ambition, helping you to commit to achieving it.

Make long-term goals specific and precise. Write down every detail as you imagine it. You will then have a clear picture of how amazing you will look and feel when you get there.

Now write down your **short-term goals**. These are the stepping stones that create a pathway to your long-term goals. Break down these goals into monthly targets. Then plan several achievements a week, and measure your progress by ticking off each success.

If you miss a goal, don't panic. Be disciplined and revise your goals regularly, reminding yourself of what you want and where you're heading.

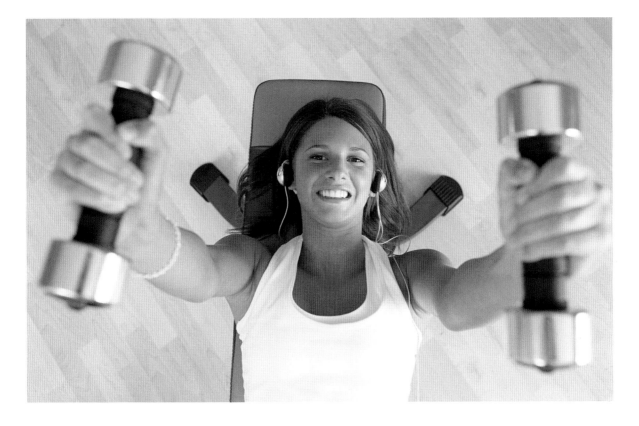

Keep a fitness diary

Writing down your daily activity helps you to chart your progress. Write down all the weights exercises you complete and your daily aerobic exercise. If your goal is weight loss, keep a food diary for a week to identify slip-ups and avoid energy slumps.

A state of mind

Try the following exercise:

- Sit quietly with no distractions. Think about a time when you felt exhausted. Remember it in detail, what you saw and what you heard. Re-live these feelings, maintaining this for about 15 seconds, then get up and think about how you feel.
- Now sit down again, and this time re-live a euphoric time when you felt empowered. Stand up and think about how you feel now.
- Compare these two emotional states and the difference you felt on standing.

This exercise shows you how your thoughts influence your physical performance.

Visualization and music

Using visualization to harness the power of the mind is undoubtedly one of the most effective ways of improving physical performance and results.

- Use visualization with each exercise: imagine the movement before you do it to achieve good technique. Remember to practise in front of a mirror (see page 18).
- Think about all the positive steps you are taking towards your goals.
- Imagine other people's praise and compliments when you achieve your goals and how fantastic that will make you feel.

Background music is another way of helping you to reach your targets. We all know how certain pieces of music fire us up, so listening to music you love while exercising helps you to experience positive thoughts and feelings, motivating you towards better results. Also allow time for relaxation, as creating joy in your life means a happier, more productive you.

Persevere with these techniques, stay focused and you will achieve results you never thought possible!

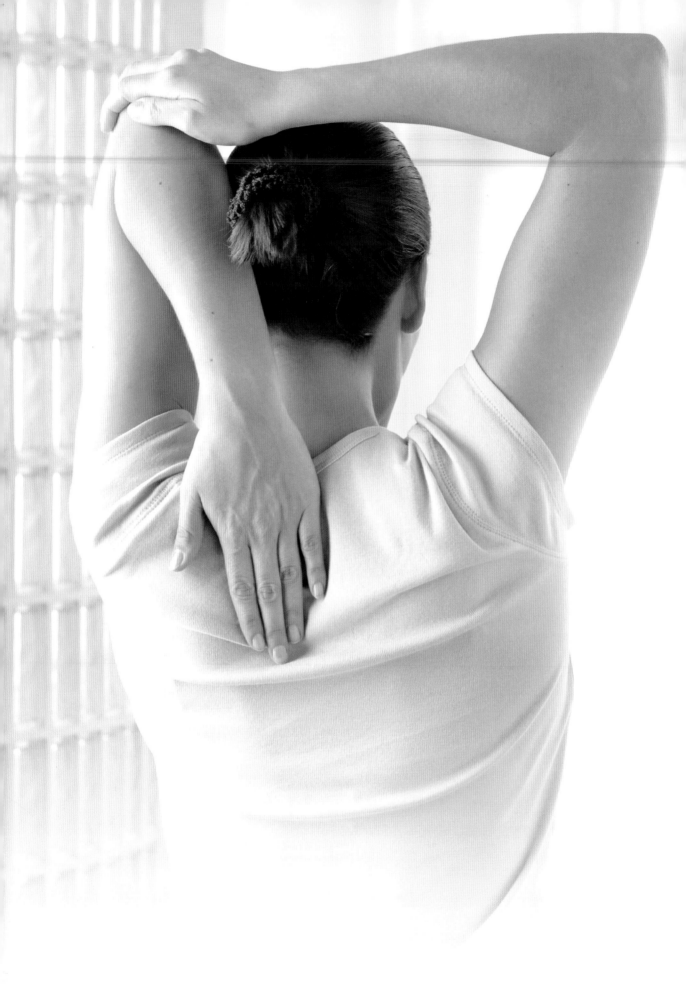

WARM-UP AND COOL-DOWN STRETCHES

warm-up/cool-down

Warming up before your workout is essential, to prepare your body for the weights exercises you are going to perform and reduce the possibility of injury. As you warm up, you raise your body's core temperature and heart rate. Blood flow increases the oxygen supply to your working muscles, making them feel more supple, and your joints become lubricated. Start with several minutes of brisk marching on the spot followed by the mobility moves on pages 25–30. This takes about 5 minutes, although some people need a longer warm-up than others.

The cool-down stretches on pages 31–39 concentrate on promoting flexibility, improving your range of motion and reducing the risk of post-exercise stiffness. Active women who stretch regularly enjoy increased energy levels and generally feel younger and more relaxed than sedentary women. One of the many benefits of regular stretching is that it helps to alleviate the aches and general stiffness associated with sedentary lifestyles and old age. Those with active lifestyles who stretch regularly enjoy unrestricted movement and generally suffer less from aches and pains.

Stretch and unwind

The cool-down stretches include some standing versions, some using a chair and some that are mat-based, so you can find the ones best suited to you. They should take around 5 minutes (or more) to complete, and will help you to relax and mentally unwind. You should stretch out each of the muscles you have used in your workout for 15–30 seconds. Ease into each stretch gradually, never use force and breathe in a relaxed manner.

Stretching helps you to relate movement to breathing. Stretching also helps you to detox by stimulating better circulation. Always stretch when you have completed your workout.

Better posture

Providing you are already warm, you can use these stretches during your daily life to promote better posture and movement with grace. Stretching releases physical and mental tension, and induces a sense of serenity and wellbeing that makes you feel refreshed and recharged.

Warming-up

Cooling down

WARMING UP
head tilts and turns

EQUIPMENT none   **REPS** 2   **SET** 1

These easy stretches help to combat tension in locked-up neck muscles. Daily stresses in your working life or long hours behind the driving wheel can cause headaches and weariness. Taking regular stretches any time you feel tension building refreshes jaded concentration, promotes mobility and makes you feel rejuvenated. Perform this stretch standing or seated.

Remember Avoid forcing the movement, turning your head only so far as to feel a comfortable stretch.

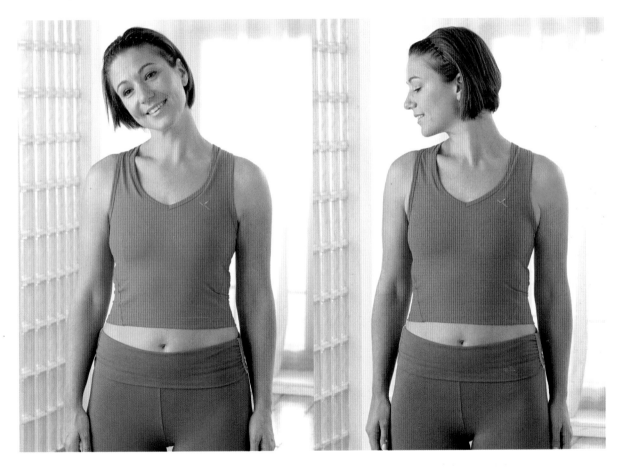

1 Maintain good posture, with your arms by your sides and your shoulders square to the front and level, and pull your navel towards your spine throughout. Tilt your right ear towards your right shoulder and hold for up to 5 seconds. Return to the start position and then repeat to the left. Breathe normally throughout.

2 From the same start position, turn your head to the right, drop your chin forward slightly and hold for up to 5 seconds. Return to the start position and then repeat to the left. Breathe normally throughout.

shoulder rolls

EQUIPMENT none   **REPS** 3–5   **SETS** 2

This movement mobilizes and loosens the muscles around the shoulders. Performed regularly, it can increase mobility and enhance postural awareness. Shoulder Rolls will encourage your chest area to open as they relax the shoulder muscles. Tense shoulders lead to poor posture, tight chest muscles and a rounded upper back. Perform this stretch standing or seated, at any time.

Remember Common places to hold tension are in the hands and the jawline, so relax them as you warm up.

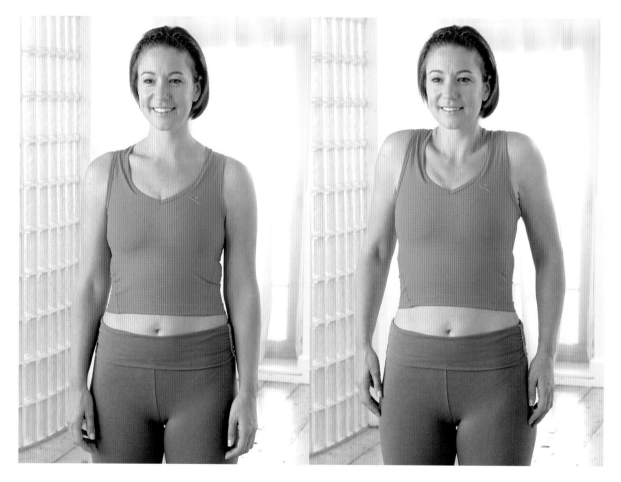

1 Maintain good posture and pull your navel towards your spine throughout. Keep your arms relaxed by your sides, with your shoulders square to the front and level. Breathe normally throughout.

2 Slowly lift and roll your shoulders back, drop them down and return to the start position. Perform 1 set. Then repeat the shoulder lift, roll your shoulders forward, drop them down and return to the start position. Perform 1 set.

trunk twist

EQUIPMENT stability ball **REPS** 6–8 **SET** 1

This rotation loosens up your spine and warms up your waist (oblique) muscles. It is also good for improving posture by helping you to get movement into your spine. Using the muscles that twist and turn your body prepares you for the core-strengthening exercises ahead, and helps you to gain postural awareness. Perform this stretch standing or seated on a stability ball.

Remember Think of your abdominal muscles wrapping around you like a corset, holding your stomach firm.

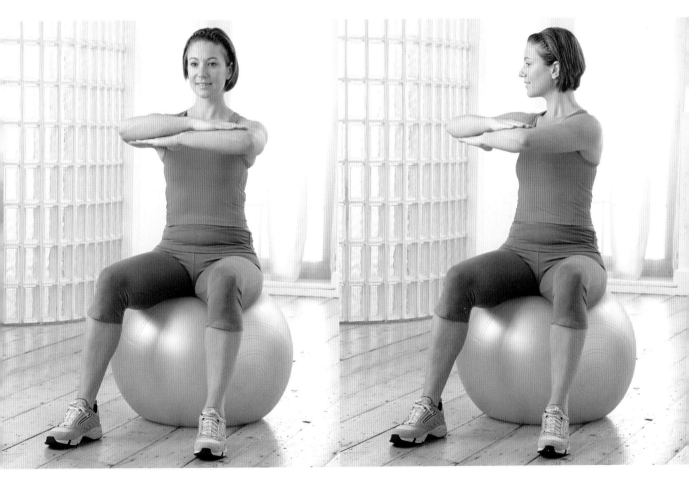

1 Maintain good posture, pull your navel towards your spine and breathe normally throughout. Place your arms one on top of the other in front of you at chest level. Lift your body weight out of your hips, keeping your hips square to the front throughout.

2 Rotate slowly to the right from your waist up, while looking towards your right elbow. Hold for 1 second and then return to the start position. Keep lifting your body weight out of your hips as you repeat to the left. Keep alternating sides.

thigh slide

EQUIPMENT none **REPS** 4 **SET** 1

This stretch is effective in helping to increase mobility in your spine, while improving body awareness and control of your central girdle as you perform the movements. Working your waist muscles in the warm-up prepares you for the weights exercises that use a similar pattern, prompting you to mentally rehearse the movements. Perform this stretch standing or seated.

Remember Keep your weight even over both feet and make sure your hips and shoulders remain facing forward.

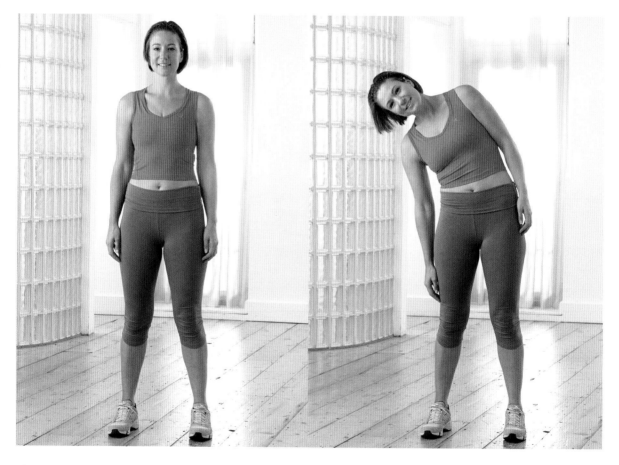

1 Stand with your feet parallel and hip-width apart, knees soft and arms relaxed by your sides. Maintain good posture and pull your navel towards your spine throughout. Look straight ahead. Make sure you do not lean forward or back. Breathe normally throughout.

2 Lift your body weight out of your hips and bend slowly to your right, sliding the palm of your right hand down your right thigh. Reach as far as is comfortable, then return to the start position. Keep lifting your body weight out of your hips as you repeat to the left. Keep alternating sides.

rock 'n' roll

EQUIPMENT none   **REPS** 4–6   **SETS 2**

These are great movements to warm and loosen your lower back, release tension and even ease back pain. Use this stretch whenever your back feels tight and fatigued. It is a relaxing movement that feels good to do, creating awareness of your pelvic positioning and helping you to prepare for the strengthening exercises ahead.

Remember Breathe normally throughout and feel the movement loosening your lower back and hips.

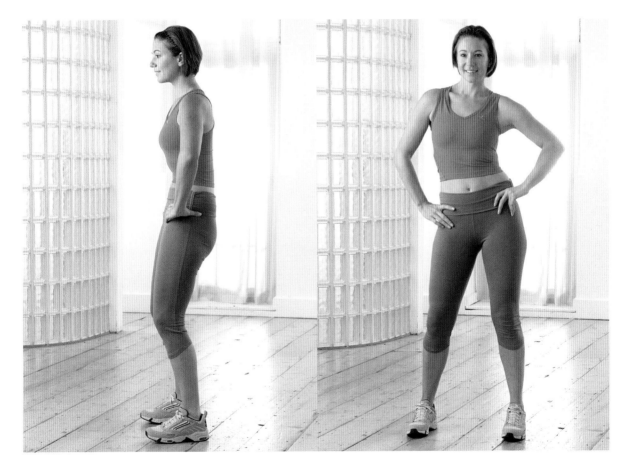

1 Maintain good posture and pull your navel towards your spine throughout. Stand with your feet hip-width apart, knees soft and hands on hips. Tilt your pelvis back (your hipbones move towards your face) then slowly uncurl your spine, returning to the start position. Repeat this rocking movement slowly, without arching your back.

2 Assuming the same start position, lengthen through your spine, taking your hips out to your left (the gap between your left rib and left hip shortens). Return to the start position and then repeat to the right.

WARM-UP AND COOL-DOWN STRETCHES **29**

knee lifts/mimic squats

EQUIPMENT none **REPS** 8 **SET** 1

Knee Lifts help to loosen the joints of your knees and improve mobility in your hips. Enhancing balance skills, they can provide an efficient way of reducing stiffness in your joints after long hours rooted to the seat of a chair. Mimic Squats also prepare your muscles and joints, taking you through a mini rehearsal in preparation for the full Squats exercise (see page 93).

Remember When performing knee lifts avoid dropping your chest towards your knee as you lift. During Mimic Squats, look straight ahead and avoid arching your back.

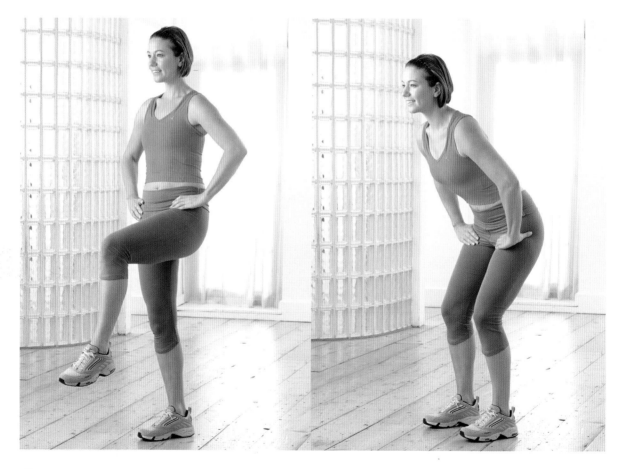

1 Maintain good posture, pull your navel towards your spine and breathe normally throughout. Stand with your feet parallel and hip-width apart, knees soft and hands on hips. Lift one foot off the floor, bending the knee and lifting it to hip height. Return to the start position and repeat on the opposite side. Keep alternating, then perform Mimic Squats.

2 Assume the same start position as for Knee Lifts. Maintain good posture, pull your navel towards your spine and breathe normally throughout. Bend your knees to 45 degrees and lean your body forward slightly at 90 degrees to your thighs. Make sure you keep your heels on the mat. Return to the start position.

calf stretch

EQUIPMENT none

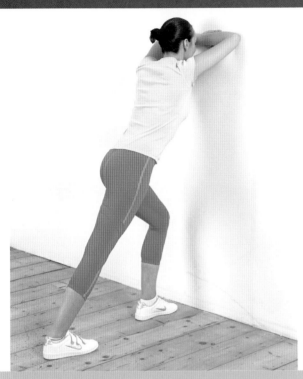

Face the wall, placing your forearms against it. Bend your left knee and position your right leg behind you, pressing your right heel into the floor, then allow your body weight to fall forward onto your arms. Keep your navel pulled towards your spine and breathe normally throughout. Hold for 15–30 seconds. Return to the start position and then repeat on the opposite side.

front of leg stretch

EQUIPMENT chair

Maintain good posture, pull your navel towards your spine and breathe normally throughout. Place your right hand on the chair back for support. Raise your left foot towards your left buttock and grasp the lifted foot with your left hand. Keeping your knees close together, lengthen up through the spine and hold for 15–30 seconds. Return to the start position and then repeat on the opposite side.

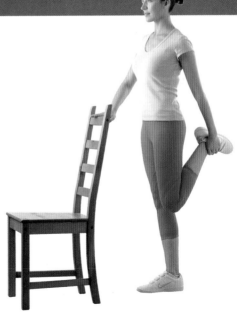

chest stretch

EQUIPMENT none

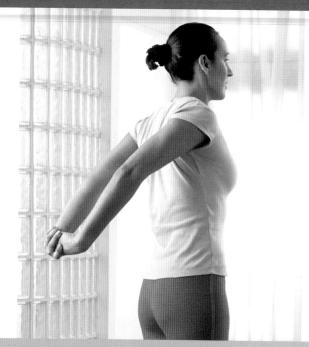

Maintain good posture, pull your navel towards your spine and breathe normally throughout. Stand with your feet parallel and hip-width apart, and your knees soft. Keep your neck and shoulders relaxed and your chin level, looking straight ahead. Clasping your hands behind your back and lifting your arms behind you, feel a stretch along the front of your chest. Hold for 15–30 seconds.

shoulder stretch

EQUIPMENT none

Maintaining good posture and pulling your navel towards your spine, bring your left arm with elbow slightly bent across your chest, placing your left hand by your right shoulder. Place your right hand on your upper left arm and gently ease the arm across your body, feeling the stretch in the back of your left shoulder. Breathe normally throughout. Hold for 15–30 seconds. Return to the start position and then repeat on the opposite side.

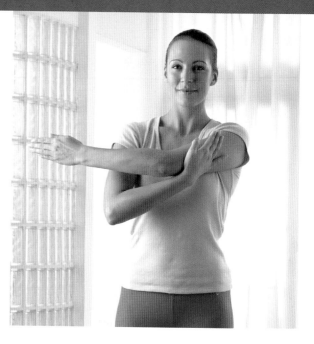

standing cat stretch

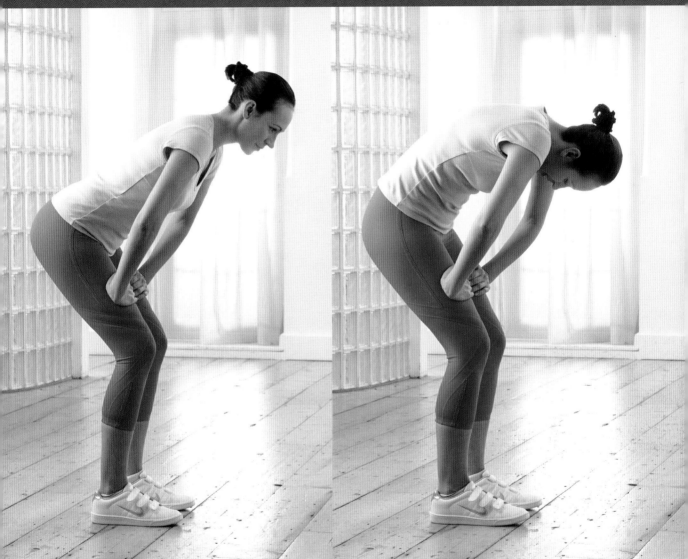

1 Standing with your feet hip-width apart and knees slightly bent, rest your palms on the fronts of your thighs. Pulling your navel towards your spine throughout, lean forward from your hips. Lengthen the back of your neck and avoid arching your back. This is your start position. Breathe in to prepare.

2 Breathing out, tilt your pelvis up (hold your abdominals firm) and drop your tailbone towards the floor, rounding your back upwards in a rippling movement until the top of your head drops forward. Your spine will form the shape of a hump-backed bridge. As you breathe in, lengthen your tailbone away from the floor, returning to the start position. Repeat.

triceps stretch

EQUIPMENT none

Stand with your feet parallel and hip-width apart, and your knees soft. Maintain good posture and pull your navel towards your spine throughout. Raise your left arm overhead and bend your left elbow, reaching down your spine with your hand. Place your right hand on your left elbow and gently pull the arm back. Feel a stretch in the back of your left arm (triceps). Breathe normally throughout. Hold for 15 seconds. Return to the start position and then repeat on the opposite side.

biceps stretch

EQUIPMENT none

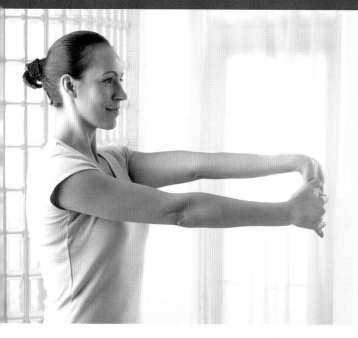

Stand with your feet parallel and hip-width apart, and your knees soft. Maintain good posture and pull your navel towards your spine throughout. Extend your left arm in front of you at shoulder level. Holding your left palm with your right hand, pull your left palm back towards you. Feel a stretch along the top of your upper arm (biceps) and from the crook of your elbow to your wrist. Breathe normally throughout. Hold for 15 seconds. Return to the start position and then repeat on the opposite side.

upper body/back stretch

EQUIPMENT chair/ledge or worktop

Use a sturdy chair back or a ledge/worktop for this stretch. Position both hands shoulder-width apart on the chair back/ledge and take a couple of steps back. Pull your navel towards your spine throughout. Keeping your knees slightly bent and hips positioned directly over your feet, allow your upper body to drop down. Breathe normally throughout. Hold for 15–30 seconds. Keep your knees bent as you come out of the stretch.

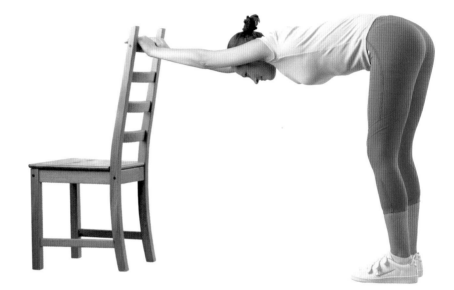

spinal rotation

EQUIPMENT armless chair

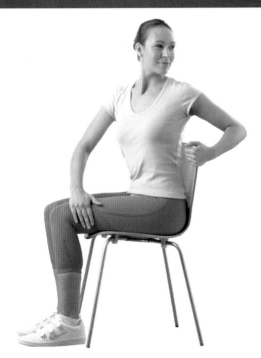

Sit on an armless chair, ensuring your knees and hips are level and your feet are flat on the floor – place a block or folded towel under your feet if necessary. Pull your navel towards your spine throughout. Place your right hand against the outside of your left thigh. Hold the back of the chair with your left hand and look over your left shoulder. Using your arms for leverage, feel a stretch down your sides. Breathe normally throughout. Hold for 15–30 seconds. Return to the start position and then repeat on the opposite side.

front of hip stretch

EQUIPMENT mat

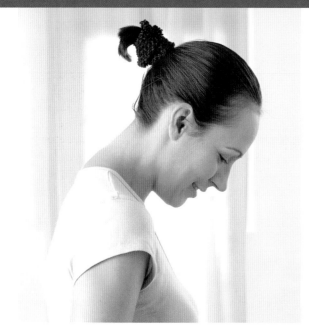

Kneel down on one knee. Pulling your navel towards your spine throughout, place your hands on the mat on either side of your leading foot and slide your back leg further out behind you. Push your hips forward until you feel a stretch in the front of the hip. (To increase the stretch, place your hands on the knee of the leading leg.) Breathe normally throughout. Hold for 15–30 seconds. Return to the start position and then repeat on the opposite side.

neck stretch

EQUIPMENT none

Perform this stretch either seated or standing. Maintain good posture, pulling your navel towards your spine, and relax your arms by your sides throughout. Lengthen up through your spine, drawing the top of your head towards the ceiling. Keep your spine neutral throughout. Lower your chin towards your chest until you feel a gentle stretch in the back of your neck and upper back. Breathe normally throughout. Hold for 5–10 seconds, then relax and repeat if you like.

side stretch

EQUIPMENT none

Stand with your feet hip-width apart and knees soft. Pull your navel towards your spine throughout and breathe normally. Extend both your arms overhead, grasping your right hand with your left, and bend slowly to the left. Use your left hand to pull your right arm gently up and over. Feel a stretch along your right side, from your arm down to your hip. Hold for 1 second, then return to the start position. Repeat on the opposite side.

hamstring stretch

EQUIPMENT chair or bench

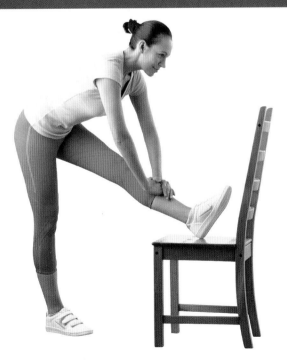

Facing the seat of a sturdy bench or chair at roughly knee height, place your left foot on the seat, keeping your supporting right leg under your hip with the knee soft. Pull your navel towards your spine and breathe normally throughout. Slowly lean forward from your hips until you feel a stretch along the back of your raised leg. Hold for 15–30 seconds. Return to the start position and then repeat on the opposite side.

buttock stretch

EQUIPMENT mat

Lie on your back with your knees bent, feet flat on the mat and hip-width apart. Breathe normally throughout. Lift your left foot and cross your left knee over your right knee. Raise your right foot off the mat, bringing the crossed knees in towards your chest and simultaneously clasping your hands over your knees. Feel a stretch in your buttocks. Hold for 15–30 seconds. Return to the start position and then repeat on the opposite side.

prone hamstring stretch

EQUIPMENT mat and scarf or towel

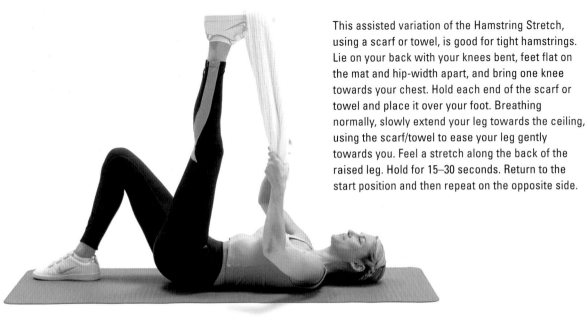

This assisted variation of the Hamstring Stretch, using a scarf or towel, is good for tight hamstrings. Lie on your back with your knees bent, feet flat on the mat and hip-width apart, and bring one knee towards your chest. Hold each end of the scarf or towel and place it over your foot. Breathing normally, slowly extend your leg towards the ceiling, using the scarf/towel to ease your leg gently towards you. Feel a stretch along the back of the raised leg. Hold for 15–30 seconds. Return to the start position and then repeat on the opposite side.

adductor stretch

EQUIPMENT mat

Sit upright, place the soles of your feet together and hold your ankles with your knees dropped out to the sides. If this position is uncomfortable and you feel your back curving, try sitting on the edge of a large cushion or rolled towel. Pull your navel towards your spine and breathe normally throughout. As you hold the position, gently press your elbows against your inner thighs. If you are more flexible, lean forward slightly from your hips while gently pressing with your elbows as before. Hold for 15–30 seconds.

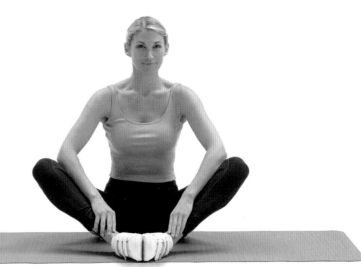

abductor stretch

EQUIPMENT mat

Sit upright on the mat with your left leg straight out in front of you. Cross your right leg over the stretched leg, positioning your right foot flat on the mat on the outside of your left knee. Place your right arm on the mat behind you for support and your left arm outside the right knee to ease the knee across your bodyline. Pull your navel towards your spine and breathe normally throughout. Feel a stretch along the outside of your thigh. Hold for 15–30 seconds. Return to the start position and then repeat on the opposite side.

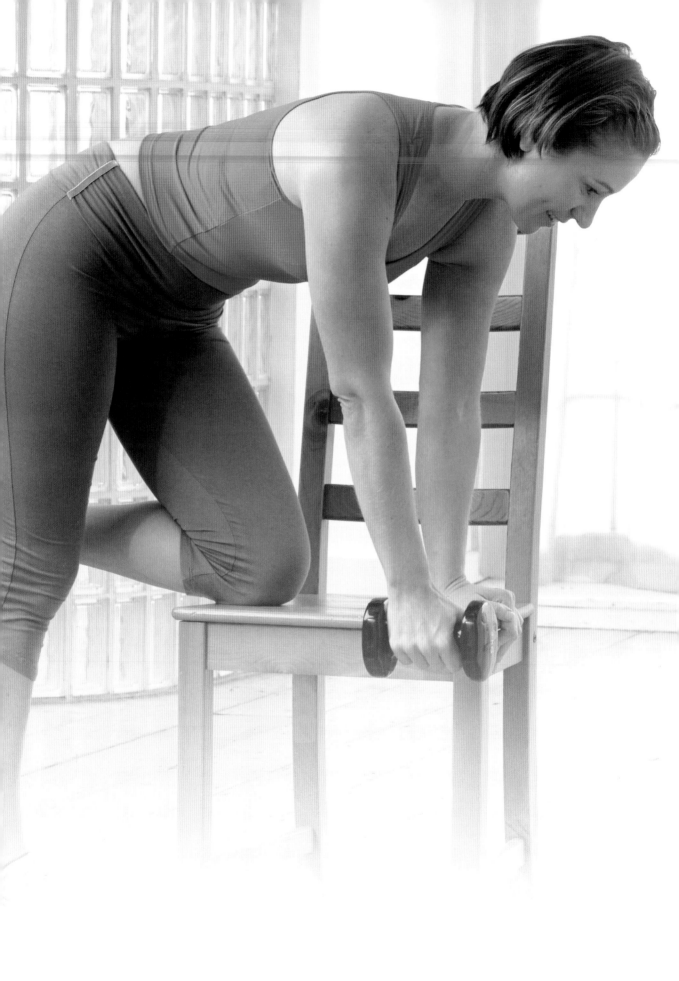

THE UPPER BODY

upper body exercises

Working with weights is the ideal way for a woman to firm, shape and strengthen her upper body. The benefits are not only reflected in your posture and overall appearance, but also have practical advantages. Everyday activities such as making beds, lifting and holding toddlers, and carrying heavy shopping, as well as heavy-duty tasks such as digging the garden or lugging the occasional suitcase around at holiday time, will become effortless. You will gain the energy, inner strength and confidence to take on new tasks and interesting leisure activities.

Be aware that upper body training is just one part of your overall balanced workout: training just one body area to the detriment of others will lead to imbalances and even injury.

Losing weight

You cannot train individual areas in isolation for weight loss, because during exercise the body is inclined to use fat from stores all over the body – including your breasts, your back and even your face! Fat loss is dependent on burning calories through physical activity.

To lose weight and burn fat efficiently, you need to combine weight training with cardiovascular workouts and eat sensibly to create a calorie deficit. If you consume more calories than your body requires for activity, they will be stored as fat.

Toning up

Toned arms and shoulders are very attractive, while firmer chest muscles improve your bust shape. A strong, shapely upper back helps to counter unattractive rounded shoulders. If you are pear-shaped, your improved upper body will draw the focus of attention away from your heavier lower half and create a more balanced appearance.

Preparation

The workout programmes (see pages 116–125) are designed for all levels. Bench-based exercises have here been replaced by versions using the stability ball, adding both variety and an excellent core challenge. Before using the stability ball, it is essential that you practise the Walkout (see page 78) and the Wheelbarrow (see page 82) for safe positioning. If this is your first introduction to working with weights, make sure you have studied pages 14–15 to enable you to select the appropriate weights for you.

Upper body exercises

chest press

EQUIPMENT mat, cushion, dumbbells   **REPS** 12–15   **SETS** 1–3

This effective exercise targets the muscles of the chest (pectoralis major), front of the shoulders (anterior deltoid) and back of the upper arms (triceps). Training the pectoral muscle that lies under the breast tissue helps to improve the shape of your bust. Select suitable weights and a large, firm cushion.

Remember Avoid bending your wrists.

1 Lie on your back with the cushion under your head and shoulders, your knees bent, and your feet flat on the mat and hip-width apart. Hold the dumbbells with your palms facing forward and bend your elbows to 90 degrees, in line with your chest. Pull your navel towards your spine throughout. Breathe in to prepare.

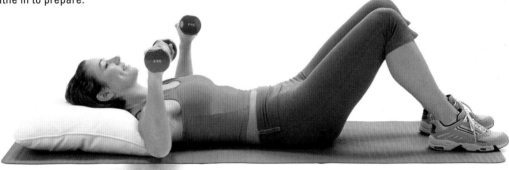

2 Breathe out and press the dumbbells towards the ceiling until your arms are nearly straight, but do not lock your elbows. Breathe in and slowly lower with control to the start position.

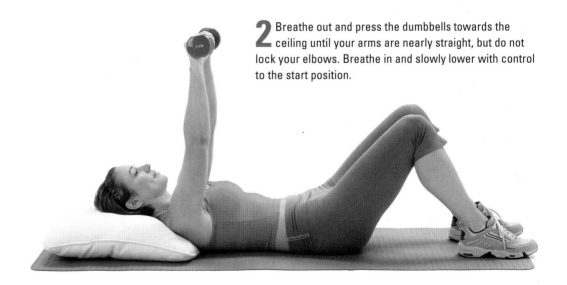

half press-up

EQUIPMENT mat, plus stability ball for variation   **REPS** 12–15   **SETS** 1–3

Press-ups work the muscles of the chest (pectoralis major), front of the shoulders (anterior deltoid) and back of the upper arms (triceps). Women generally do not practise exercises that use their own body weight because their wrists are weaker, and therefore they tend to find them difficult. The Half Press-up is a more comfortable version that needs no special equipment and can be performed almost anywhere.

Remember As your arms start to fatigue, ensure you maintain a straight body line. Avoid lifting up your buttocks or letting your stomach drop.

1 Kneel on all fours with your shoulders over your wrists, hands slightly wider than shoulder-width apart and fingertips pointing forward. Walk your hands forward, allowing your body weight to shift onto your arms. From here on, your body should remain in a straight line from shoulders to knees with your neck in line with your spine. Hold your abdominals strongly, pulling your navel towards your spine throughout.

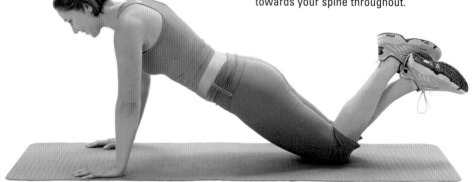

2 Breathe in, bend your elbows sideways and lower your chest towards the mat (if you find this difficult, do not bend your elbows so far). Breathe out and press back up to the start position, taking care not to raise your eye line.

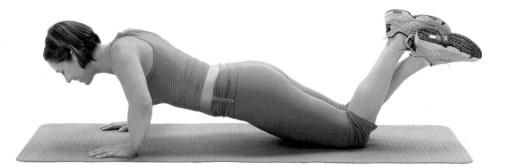

variation

Many women prefer stability ball press-ups to conventional full press-ups, as they add a balance challenge to the exercise. The further you walk your hands away from the ball, the greater the intensity. To increase the emphasis on your chest area, place your hands slightly further apart. Practising the Wheelbarrow (see page 82) first will equip you with sound technique in preparation for ball press-ups.

Remember Avoid pulling your body weight back towards the ball and allowing the ball to roll backwards.

1 Begin with your stomach on the ball. Walk your hands forward until your thighs rest on the ball and your body forms a straight line from your heels to your shoulders. Position your hands under your shoulders with your fingertips pointing forward. Hold your abdominals firm throughout. Keep your shoulder blades anchored and your neck in line with your spine.

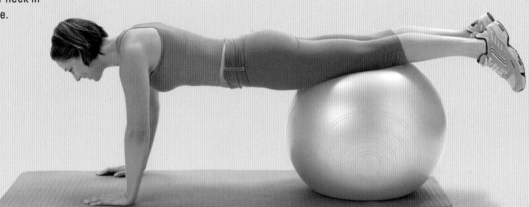

2 Breathe in and slowly bend your elbows to 90 degrees as you lower your chest towards the mat, keeping your stomach and thighs firm and your legs straight. Breathe out and press back up to the start position.

pec flyes

EQUIPMENT mat, cushion, dumbbells **REPS** 12–15 **SETS** 1–3

This exercise targets muscles of the chest (pectoralis major) and front of the shoulders (anterior deltoid). Working these muscles in a horizontal position means that when you return the weights to the start position, the muscular tension diminishes. To achieve good results you must concentrate mostly on the first half of each repetition, allowing a gentle stretch as your arms open at the bottom. Select suitable weights and a large, firm cushion.

Remember Avoid bending your wrists.

1 Lie on your back with the cushion under your head and shoulders, your knees bent, and your feet flat on the mat and hip-width apart. Hold a dumbbell in each hand and extend your arms above your chest with your elbows slightly bent – imagine hugging a tree – and palms facing each other. Keep your shoulder blades anchored and pull your navel towards your spine throughout. Look straight up.

2 Breathe in and carry your arms outwards until they are almost parallel with the floor, keeping your elbows slightly bent. Hold for 1 second and feel a gentle stretch across your chest and shoulders. Then breathe out and bring your arms towards each other again, feeling your chest muscles contracting on the effort.

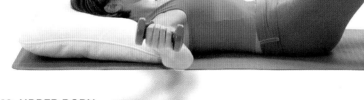

dumbbell pullovers

EQUIPMENT stability ball, dumbbell   **REPS** 12–15   **SETS** 1–3

This movement works the large back muscle (latissimus dorsi) by using an arc-shaped movement that also activates muscles known as the serrati, which help to pull the shoulder blade forward and rotate it, and also pull down the lower ribs. Used regularly, this exercise will help to give your back a wonderful shape because of the large area this muscle covers. Select one heavier weight and a stability ball. Practise the Walkout (see page 78) first.

Remember Contract your buttocks throughout to avoid dropping your hips.

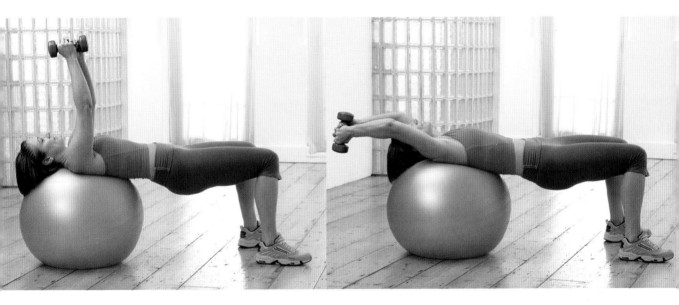

1 Lie back on the ball with your head, neck, shoulders and back supported. Hold the dumbbell in both hands and raise it directly above your head at eye level, with your elbows slightly bent. Pull your navel towards your spine throughout.

2 Breathing in, draw your shoulder blades down and lower the dumbbell behind your head as far as you feel comfortable, feeling the stretch in your outer mid-back area. Feel your back muscles contracting as you breathe out and smoothly return to the start position.

sky diver

EQUIPMENT mat   **REPS** 10–12   **SETS** 1–2

Gaining strength in the lower half of the upper back muscle (trapezius) and the smaller muscles situated on either side of the spine (rhomboids) is vital to help improve posture and create muscular balance. These muscles are attached to the shoulder blades, so improved strength in this area can help to prevent injuries and improve the way you hold yourself.

Remember Once the movement feels easy, practise it with light dumbbells.

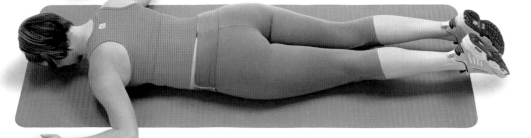

1 Lie face down with your forehead resting on the mat. Bring your arms out to your sides and bend your elbows at 90 degrees, with your palms flat and fingertips pointing forward. Keep your legs together and parallel. Breathe in to prepare.

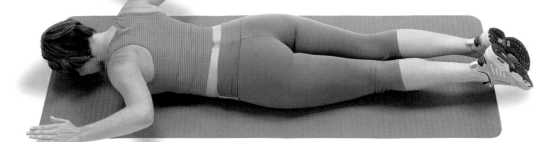

2 Breathe out, initiating the movement by gently squeezing your shoulder blades back and down, and lift your arms off the mat. Keep your forehead on the mat. Hold for 2–3 seconds, breathing normally, and then lower back to the start position.

upward row

EQUIPMENT dumbbells **REPS** 12–15 **SET** 1

The rowing action of this exercise places emphasis on the middle part of your shoulders (medial deltoids), activates the supporting muscles of your upper back (trapezius) and works the front of your arms (biceps). As part of a varied workout, Upward Row will strengthen this vulnerable area, making it easier to carry shopping and lift babies. It will also help you to achieve eye-catching definition across your shoulders. Select suitable weights.

Remember Relax your shoulders so that they don't lift up with the dumbbells.

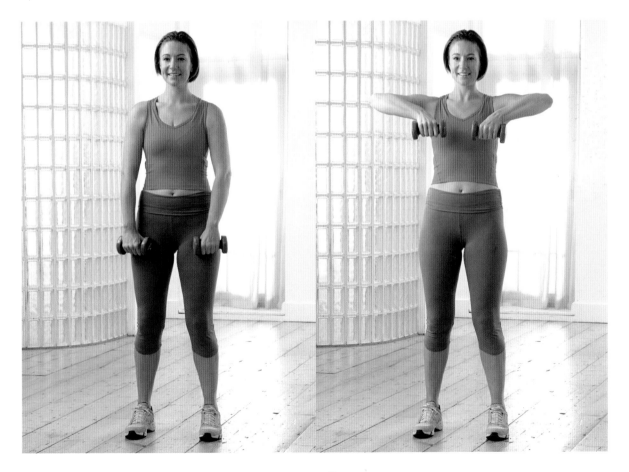

1 Stand with your feet hip-width apart and your knees soft. Maintain good posture and pull your navel towards your spine throughout. Hold a dumbbell in each hand and position your arms shoulder-width apart with your palms facing the front of your thighs. Breathe in to prepare.

2 Leading the movement with your elbows, breathe out and lift the dumbbells up to chest level. Keep them close to your body line and always lower than your elbows. Breathe in and slowly lower the dumbbells to the start position.

single-arm row

EQUIPMENT chair, dumbbell **REPS** 12–15 **SETS** 1–3

This exercise works the large muscles of the mid-back (latissimus dorsi), the smaller back muscles (rhomboids) and also the front of the arms (biceps). Strengthening the mid-back muscles develops a sleek, hourglass shape, creating a more defined waist and the illusion of slender hips. For keen sportswomen, strength in the back is essential. It will also improve your posture and help to protect against injury. You will need a sturdy chair and a suitable weight.

Remember Concentrate on using your back muscles, drawing the shoulder blade of the working arm towards your spine as the elbow lifts.

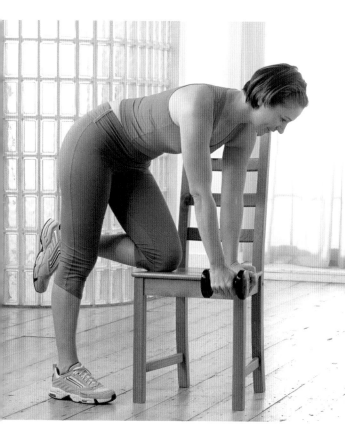
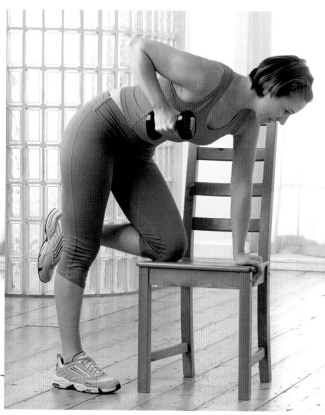

1 Place your left knee on the chair, with your left hand in front of you on the seat for stability. Your right foot remains under your right hip. Hold a dumbbell in your right hand with your arm hanging down towards floor. Pull your navel towards your spine throughout, and keep your back straight and shoulders relaxed and parallel to the seat. Breathe in to prepare.

2 Breath out and, leading with your elbow and keeping your wrist straight, draw the dumbbell up towards the side of your ribcage, feeling your back muscles contracting. Slowly lower with control to the start position. Perform the required number of reps and then repeat on the opposite side.

two-arm row

EQUIPMENT dumbbells **REPS** 12–15 **SETS** 1–3

The Two-Arm Row targets the same muscles in your back as the Single-Arm Row, but this version requires more effort because your back and stomach have to stabilize and support you as you lean forward. Your efforts will be rewarded with less bra-strap fat, and a beautifully svelte back. Select suitable weights.

Remember Feel your shoulder blades moving closer together as you lift the dumbbells upwards.

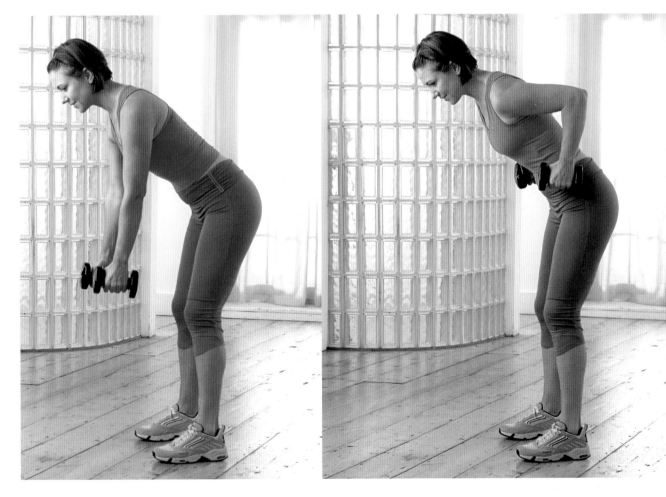

1 Hold a dumbbell in each hand. Stand with your feet hip-width apart, knees slightly bent and arms by your sides with palms facing in. Pulling your navel towards your spine throughout, lean forward from your hips, allowing your arms to hang down from your shoulders. Keep your eye line towards the mat. Breathe in to prepare

2 Breathe out and pull the dumbbells up towards your waist, bending both elbows to 90 degrees. Hold for 1 second, then breathe in and slowly lower the dumbbells to the start position.

shoulder press

EQUIPMENT chair, dumbbells **REPS** 12–15 **SETS** 1–3

This is a fantastic exercise that works the shoulder muscles (deltoids) and many other supporting muscles in this area, as well as the backs of the arms (triceps). Women are generally weaker in these areas. The multiple gains from this exercise include being able to lift heavy objects into overhead storage and firming up the wobbly area at the backs of your arms. Select light weights initially, as your supporting muscles will be working hard to stabilize you.

Remember For a further challenge try this standing up, or sitting on the stability ball.

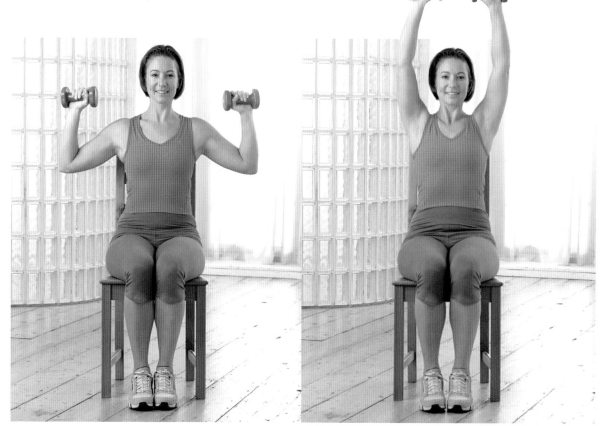

1 Sit on the edge of the chair with your feet flat on the floor. Hold a dumbbell in each hand and bring the weights to shoulder level, with your palms facing forward and dumbbells parallel to the floor. Hold your abdominals firmly, pulling your navel towards your spine, and maintain good posture throughout. Breathe in to prepare.

2 Breathe out and push the dumbbells up, raising your arms above your head. Keep the dumbbells slightly in front of your head when your arms are extended and avoid locking your elbows. Breathe in and slowly lower the dumbbells to the start position.

lateral raise

EQUIPMENT dumbbells **REPS** 12–15 **SETS** 1–3

The definitive exercise for targeting the mid-shoulders (medial deltoids), this movement creates great shape and definition and balances your proportions, creating the illusion of a smaller waist. Stronger shoulders will help with lifting and carrying, enabling you to go about everyday tasks with poise and confidence. Select suitable weights.

Remember Start practising this with lighter weights and make sure you avoid tension by consciously relaxing your shoulders.

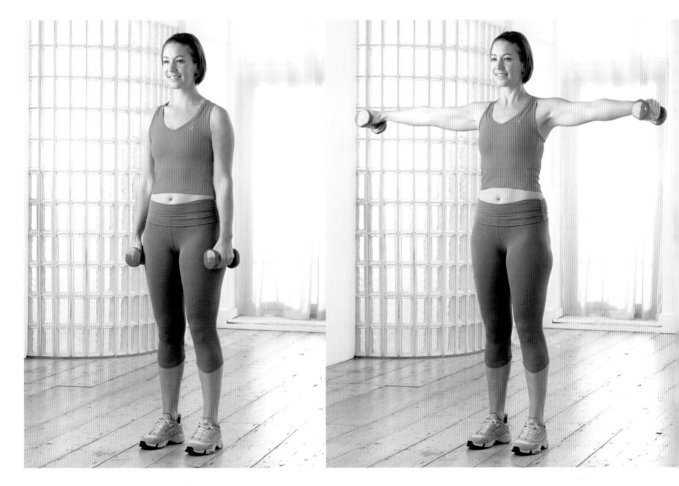

1 Stand with your feet hip-width apart and knees soft. Maintain good posture and pull your navel towards your spine throughout. Hold a dumbbell in each hand with your arms by your sides, palms facing in and elbows slightly bent. Breathe in to prepare.

2 Breathe out and slowly raise your arms out to the sides with elbows slightly bent, until the dumbbells reach shoulder level. Your forearms and palms will be facing the floor. Hold for 1 second, then breathe in and slowly lower to the start position.

shoulder shaper

EQUIPMENT stability ball/chair, dumbbells **REPS** 12–15 **SETS** 1–3

Add variety, challenge and intensity to your routine with this exercise that works the shoulder muscles (deltoids) and improves coordination. Your postural muscles work hard in this variation. This provides stability for your torso and helps you to avoid leaning away from the weights. Select lighter dumbbells.

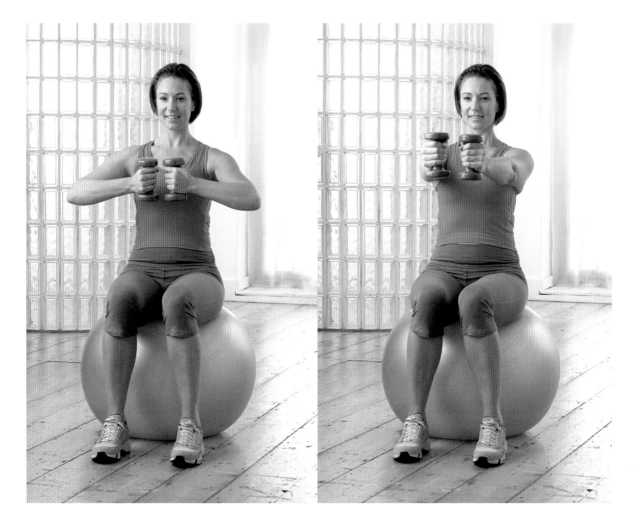

1 Sit upright on the chair or stability ball with your feet flat on the floor and a comfortable distance apart, and your knees over your heels. Maintain good posture and pull your navel in towards your spine throughout. Hold a dumbbell in each hand in front of you at chest level, bending your elbows out to the sides with your palms facing towards you.

2 Breathe in and smoothly extend your arms in front of you at chest level, so that your palms are now facing each other and the dumbbells pointing down towards the floor. Avoid locking your elbows. Lengthen up through your spine, drawing the top of your head towards the ceiling.

Remember This movement may prove tiring to begin with, so build up the reps gradually. Stop if your muscles fatigue or you will lose technique.

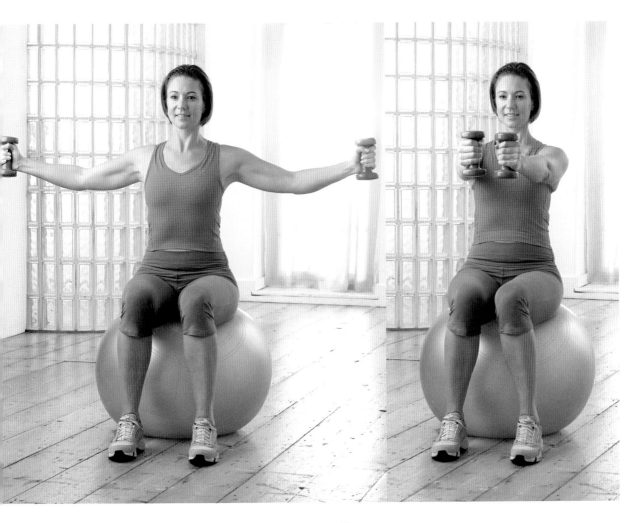

3 Breathe out and carry the weights out to the sides. Keep your arms level and parallel to the floor. Your palms are now facing forward with the dumbbells still pointing down towards the floor. Relax your shoulders.

4 Breathe in and bring your arms back in front of you so that they are now extended with your palms facing each other. Breathe out and bend your elbows out to the sides, returning the dumbbells to the start position in front of your chest.

cuff rotator

EQUIPMENT mat, cushion, dumbbell, towel **REPS** 12–15 **SETS** 1–2

This is an excellent exercise for strengthening the group of muscles that are collectively called the rotator cuff muscles. These deep shoulder muscles help to maintain joint stability by holding the head of the upper arm in the correct position. Strengthening the rotator group effectively helps to guard against potential injury. You will need a small cushion and a folded towel. Select a very light weight.

Remember If this movement creates tension in your neck, practise it without a dumbbell.

1 Lie on your side on the mat with your hips stacked and knees bent forward at 45 degrees to your body. Place a small cushion between your head and arm for good neck-to-spine alignment. Position a folded towel between your elbow and side, and anchor your elbow at the side of your waist. Hold the dumbbell, keeping your palm facing the floor.

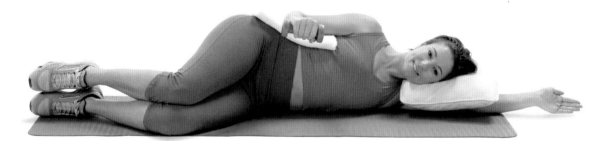

2 Breathe in to prepare, pull your navel towards your spine, then breathe out and draw your shoulder blade in towards your back as you rotate the dumbbell up through 90 degrees. Hold for 1 second, then breathe in and return to the start position. Perform the required number of reps and then repeat on the opposite side.

rear lifts

EQUIPMENT dumbbells   **REPS** 12–15   **SETS** 1–3

Focusing on the backs of your shoulders (posterior deltoids) and upper arms (triceps), these lifts firm and sculpt that hard-to-reach flabby area everyone apart from you can see! Rear Lifts will also add definition to the back of your arms, an area prone to losing muscle tone. Select suitable weights.

Remember Try not to let your ribs 'pop out', and avoid tilting forward as you press the weights behind you.

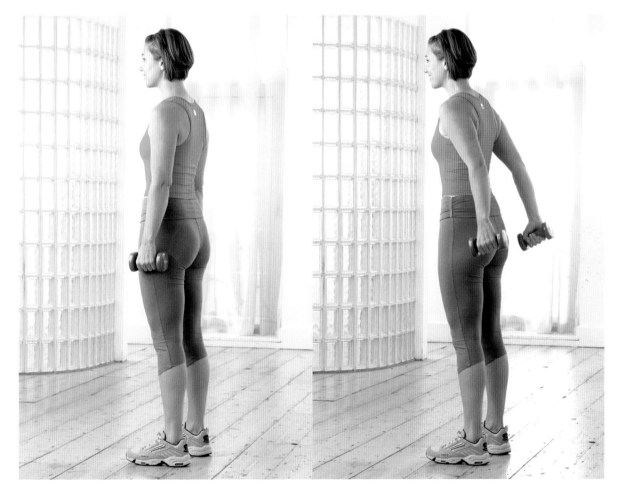

1 Stand with your feet hip-width apart and knees soft. Maintain good posture and pull your navel towards your spine throughout. Hold a dumbbell in each hand, with your arms by your sides and your palms facing in. Lengthen up through your spine, drawing the top of your head towards the ceiling. Breathe in to prepare.

2 Breathe out and press your arms back in a straight line as far as you can, keeping your shoulders down. Gently squeeze your shoulder blades together at the top of the movement and hold for 1 second. Breathe in and slowly lower to the start position.

sky reach

EQUIPMENT mat, dumbbells **REPS** 8–12 **SETS** 1–3

This is a simple but amazingly effective movement that exercises the muscles responsible for holding your shoulder blades in the correct position (subscapularis and serratus anterior). If your shoulder blades tend to stick out like chicken wings on your upper back, this indicates an underlying weakness in the musculature of this area and therefore a greater propensity for bad posture and shoulder injury. Select lighter weights. (If you are starting the Essential Workout on page 118, practise without weights.)

Remember Imagine you are making an imprint of your dumbbells on the ceiling as you push them upwards.

1 Lie on your back with your knees bent, and your feet flat on the mat and hip-width apart. Hold a dumbbell in each hand above your chest, with your palms facing each other. Reach both arms towards the ceiling so that the dumbbells are positioned directly over your chest. Gently squeeze your shoulder blades back so that they are flat on the mat. Breathe in to prepare.

2 Breathe out as you push the dumbbells up towards the ceiling, making sure that your elbows are straight as you do so. Breathe in and slowly lower to the start position.

biceps beautifier

EQUIPMENT dumbbells   **REPS** 12–15   **SETS** 1–3

The muscles that shape the fronts of your upper arms (biceps) need sculpting to look good in sleeveless tops. This exercise provides results quickly and helps to give your arms desirable shape and lean definition. Developing strength in your upper arms also means you can take everyday activities in your stride. Select suitable weights.

Remember Keep your back still and maintain control of your movements – never let momentum carry you through.

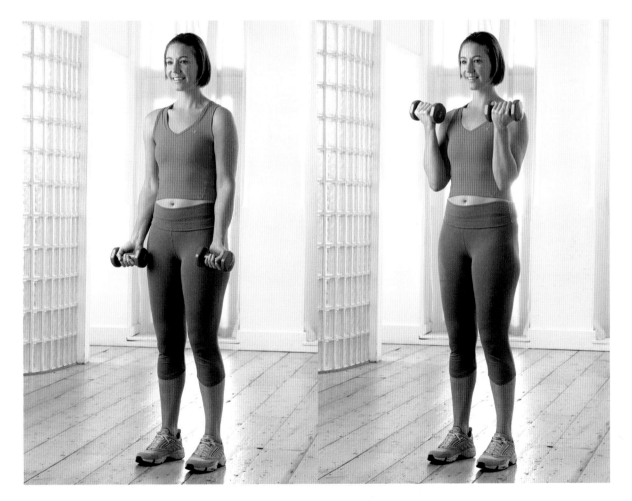

1 Stand with your feet hip-width apart and knees soft. Maintain good posture and pull your navel towards your spine throughout. Hold the dumbbells with your palms facing forward and arms by your sides with elbows slightly bent. Breathe in to prepare.

2 Breathe out, keeping your elbows close to your body as you lift the dumbbells up to your shoulders. Squeeze your biceps at the end of the curl, then breathe in and slowly lower to the start position.

hammer curl

EQUIPMENT dumbbells, plus stability ball for variation   **REPS** 12–15   **SETS** 1–3

This variation of the basic Biceps Beautifier (see page 59) is a valuable exercise as it works on defining and sculpting the outer part of your upper arms (biceps). It will help to create an illusion of longer, leaner arms because it shapes the outermost area of the biceps. Select suitable weights.

Remember Keep your body still when lifting the weights.

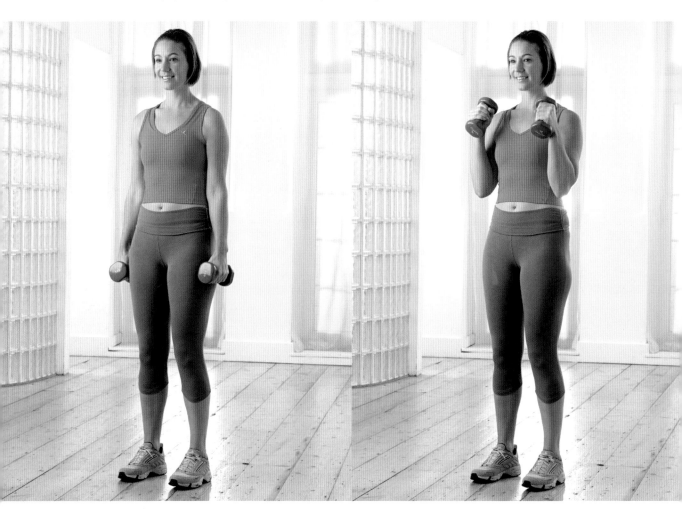

1 Stand with your feet hip-width apart and knees soft. Maintain good posture and pull your navel towards your spine throughout. Hold a dumbbell in each hand with your arms close to your sides, palms facing in and elbows slightly bent. Breathe in to prepare.

2 Keeping your elbows close to your sides, breathe out and lift the dumbbells towards your shoulders. Squeeze your biceps at the end of the curl, then breathe in and slowly lower to the start position.

variation

This challenging variation allows you to continue practising either of the biceps exercises (see pages 59 and 60) using the stability ball to further enhance your balance and core strength. The Hammer Curl has been shown here, but you can use the Biceps Beautifier version to add variety. Select suitable weights.

Remember This exercise will fatigue your supporting leg, so lift your body weight up and out of the supporting hip throughout and be sure to switch legs after 8 reps on one side.

Stand with the stability ball in front of you, holding a dumbbell in each hand. Place your left foot on top of the ball and stand firmly on your right foot. Pull your navel in towards your spine and hold your body still throughout. Avoid sinking into your supporting hip. Keep your arms close to your sides, palms facing in. Breathe in to prepare, then breathe out and perform the Hammer Curl (see step 2 opposite). Perform a maximum of 8 reps and then repeat on the opposite side.

triceps toner

EQUIPMENT chair, dumbbell, plus medicine ball for variation **REPS** 12–15 **SETS** 1–3

The backs of the upper arms (triceps) is an area many women dislike about their bodies as fat easily accumulates here. This excellent exercise shapes and tones these muscles, so that you will soon be able to wave with confidence! You can do this exercise standing, or sitting on a sturdy chair (as shown) for an enhanced technique. Select a suitable weight.

Remember Keep your upper arm still and do not allow your elbow to drift outwards.

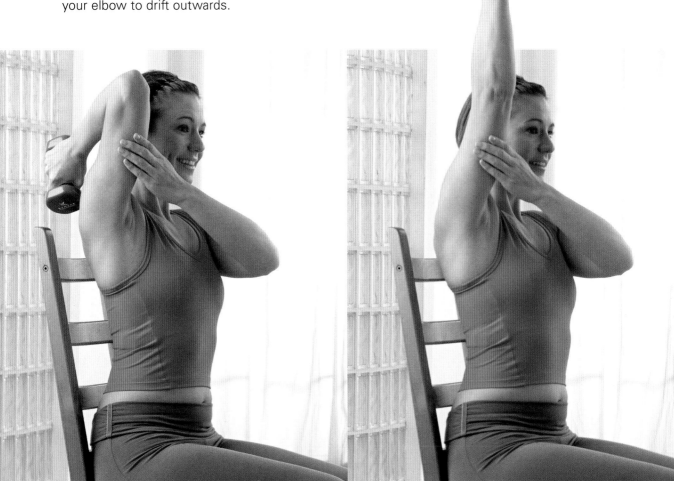

1 Sit upright and pull your navel towards you spine throughout. Hold the dumbbell in one hand behind your head, keeping your elbow level with your head. Use the opposite hand to support the back of your arm and maintain good alignment. Breathe in to prepare.

2 Breathe out and slowly push the dumbbell up towards the ceiling. Keep your elbow close to your head as you extend your arm. Breathe in and slowly lower to the start position. Perform the required number of reps and then repeat on the opposite side.

variation

This is a highly effective variation using a medicine ball. Select a 2 kg (4½ lb) medicine ball to begin with. The exercise can be performed in a seated position as before, or standing.

Remember Look straight ahead and keep your shoulder blades down.

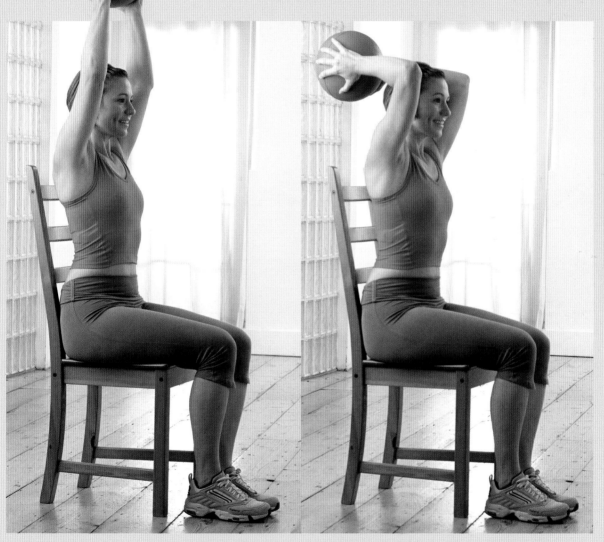

1 Sit with your feet hip-width apart and knees soft. Place your hands on either side of the ball and hold it directly above your head. Keep your shoulders, elbows and wrists in line with each other and look straight ahead. Maintain good posture, pull your navel towards your spine and hold your body still throughout.

2 Breathe in as you slowly lower the ball behind your head, keeping your elbows still. Breathe out and slowly extend your arms to return to the start position.

french press

EQUIPMENT mat, dumbbells **REPS** 12–15 **SETS** 1–3

This exercise isolates and sculpts the muscles at the backs of the upper arms (triceps). Wobbly upper arms are ageing and fat quickly accumulates here, so this area is one of women's prime 'target zones'. This movement is an excellent overall exercise that helps to create great shape. Select suitable weights.

Remember Do not allow your elbows to drift in or out to the side.

1 Lie on your back with knees bent, and feet flat on the mat and hip-width apart. Hold a dumbbell in each hand, point your elbows towards the ceiling and, bending your elbows to 90 degrees, position the dumbbells by your head. Breathe in to prepare.

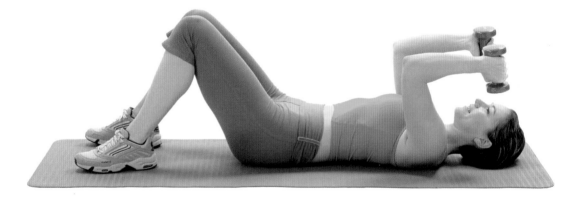

2 Keeping your upper arms stable, breathe out and push the dumbbells slowly up towards the ceiling, so that your arms extend above your head. Avoid locking your elbows. Breathe out and slowly lower to the start position, bending your elbows to 90 degrees.

dips

EQUIPMENT chair   **REPS** 12–15   **SETS** 1–3

Using your own body weight makes Dips a versatile exercise that can be done anywhere without using weights. Practising this exercise concentrates on the area at the backs of the upper arms (triceps). Dips also help to perfect your posture and will improve strength and upper arm shape. You will need a sturdy chair or bench.

Remember Avoid this exercise if you have wrist problems.

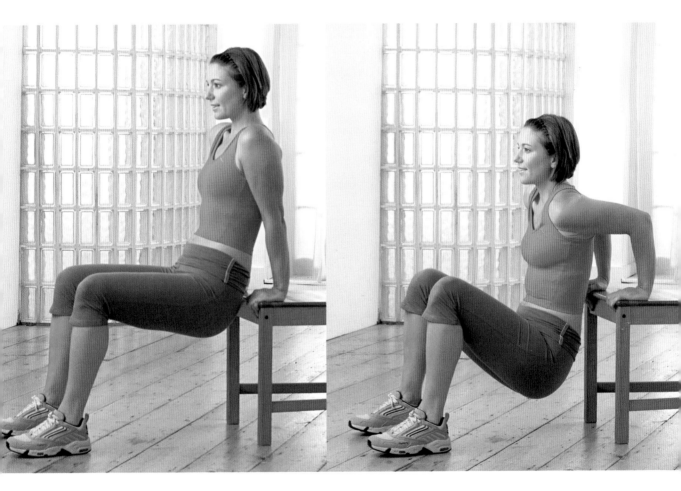

1 Sit on the edge of the chair or bench. Position your feet hip-width apart and flat on the floor, knees bent at 90 degrees and your heels slightly beyond your knees. Place your hands on the edge of the chair with fingertips pointing forward. Transfer your body weight off the chair without locking your elbows. Keep your back close to the seat and straight.

2 Pull your navel towards your spine and keep your shoulder blades down throughout. Breathe in and lower yourself down, with your arms bending to 90 degrees and elbows pointing back. Breathe out and slowly push back up to the start position.

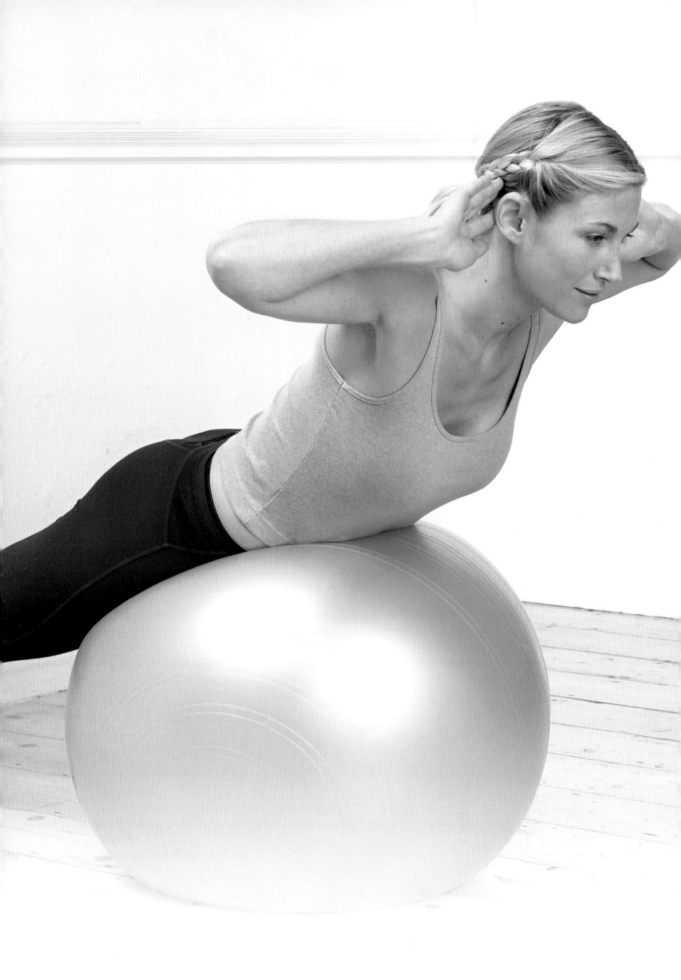

THE MID-SECTION BODY

abdominals and back

Strengthening the muscles that help you to maintain good posture will not only make you stand tall, look slimmer, and create poise and elegance, but will also have an amazing effect on your self-esteem. Training the deep muscles that provide support to your spine and help you to hold your stomach in will reward you with a strong, conditioned back that is injury resistant and resilient, together with a toned, firm stomach that will support your lower back and look great!

With good posture you will be able to achieve sound technique, which is essential in lifting weights and maintaining a healthy, pain-free back.

A balanced progression
The exercises in this section are carefully structured to form the cornerstone of your weights workout. The complete mid-section is chosen with a balanced approach in mind, and is designed to suit different levels in order to provide a continuing challenge for your body and mind as you progress. The basic foundation movements incorporated into the Essential Workout (see page 118) are aimed at improving your posture and self-awareness and will get you off to a flying start.

Working the abdomen
A variety of abdominal exercises that use different start positions are included, some of which employ the stability ball to enhance the training effect. Use the visualization techniques you learned earlier (see pages 20–21) to help you to achieve good results when performing each exercise and to concentrate fully on the muscles that are doing the work. Practise the Walkout (see page 78) and the Wheelbarrow (see page 82) before attempting any stability ball exercises.

Working the back
The back exercises complement the abdominal workouts to help you to gain and maintain a strong, flexible and healthy spine, and eliminate postural weaknesses such as an over-hollow back or rounded shoulders. The overall result will help to eradicate back pain, make you appear taller and more slender, and take years off your looks!

Abdominals and back

pelvic tilts

EQUIPMENT mat, foam ball **REPS** 10–12 **SETS** 1–2

Pelvic Tilts are easy to do and are effective in strengthening and firming the lower abdominal area (transversus abdominis). Great for the muscles of the pelvic floor (pubococcygeus), they will also help if you suffer from weakness in this area. In addition, this is an excellent exercise for a weak lower back, and will firm your buttocks and thighs. You will need a foam ball.

Remember Roll up only as far as you are comfortable, using your abdominals to control the movement.

1 Lie on your back with your knees bent, feet flat on the mat and hip-width apart, and holding a foam ball between your knees. Position your heels a comfortable distance from your buttocks, placing your arms at your sides with your palms facing down. Breathe in to prepare.

2 Breathe out, lift your pelvic floor and pull your navel towards your spine, and squeeze firmly on the foam ball. Gently squeeze your buttocks as you slowly curl your tailbone up and peel your spine off the mat. Stop when there is a straight line between your upper back and knees. Breathe in and hold for 1 second, then breathe out and slowly uncurl to the start position.

supawoman

EQUIPMENT mat, towel (no towel for variation)   **REPS** 12–15   **SETS** 1–3

An essential exercise for the lower back, this movement helps to strengthen the muscles that run the length of your spine (spinal extensors) and provide support and stability in the lower back. Practised regularly, it can also help to prevent lower back pain and improve your posture. You will need a folded towel for head comfort.

Remember Think of lengthening the top of your head away from your tailbone as you lift your arm and leg, and keep your hips pressed down.

1 Lie on your front, resting your forehead on a folded towel for good alignment. Stretch both arms in front of you, with palms facing down, and relax your neck. Position your legs slightly apart and straight. Pull your navel towards your spine and keep your shoulder blades pulled down throughout.

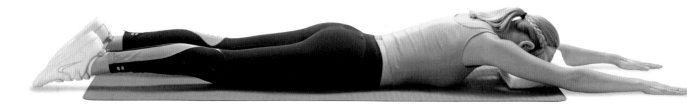

2 Breathe in as you lift your left arm and right leg, keeping your head on the towel. Hold for 1 second, then breathe out and slowly lower to the start position. Repeat on the opposite side. Keep alternating sides.

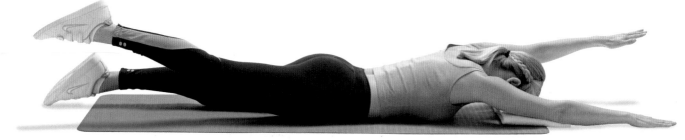

variation

The kneeling variation of the basic Supawoman exercise is more intense and requires good core control. It provides an excellent progression from the lying-down basic exercise by challenging your spinal extensors, balance and co-ordination.

Remember Think of reaching your fingertips away from your toes as you lift your arm and leg.

1 Kneel on all fours with your shoulders directly over your hands and your hips over your knees. Keep your head and neck aligned with your spine, pull your navel towards your spine and ensure you keep your shoulder blades pulled down throughout.

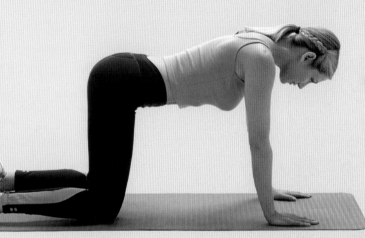

2 Breathing in, lift and extend your left arm and right leg so that they are parallel to the floor. Keep your hips and shoulders square to the floor. Hold for 1 second, then breathe out and slowly lower to the start position. Repeat on the opposite side. Keep alternating sides.

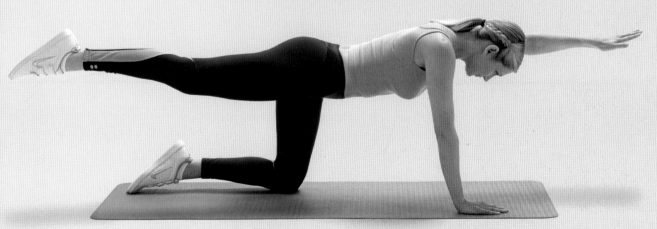

spine extension

EQUIPMENT stability ball, plus dumbbell for variation   **REPS** 12–15   **SET** 1

Exercising your mid- and lower back (erector spinae) and your buttocks (gluteals) with Spine Extensions on the stability ball is the perfect way to help you achieve core stability and correct posture. Strengthening your lower back can also help to prevent lower back pain. You will need a clear wall space against which to brace your feet.

Remember Pull your shoulder blades down throughout the movement.

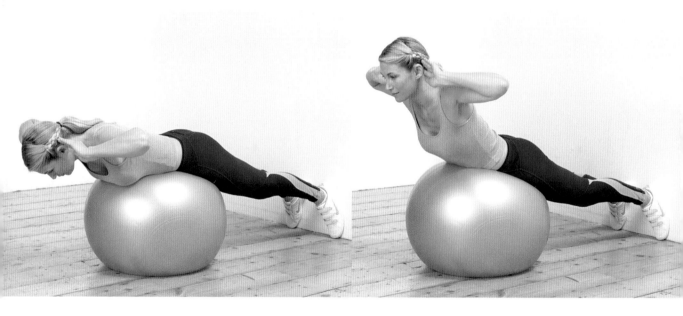

1 Lie with your stomach and hips on the ball, bracing your feet against the join of the floor and wall. Your chest, neck and head should be off the ball, with your head lower than your hips, and your hands positioned beside your head. Breathe in to prepare.

2 Breathe out, pull your navel towards your spine, and contract your buttock and back muscles as you raise your upper body. Your shoulders, hips and knees should form a line. Hold for 1 second, then breathe in and slowly lower to the start position.

variation

This variation is more difficult because it uses a weight to increase the intensity of the lift. Working the upper and lower back (erector spinae) shoulders (scapular stabilizers), buttocks (gluteals) and numerous abdominal muscles, this provides an extra challenge to the regular Spine Extension on the ball. Select one heavier weight.

Remember Think of lengthening the top of your head away from your tailbone and keep your shoulder blades down throughout.

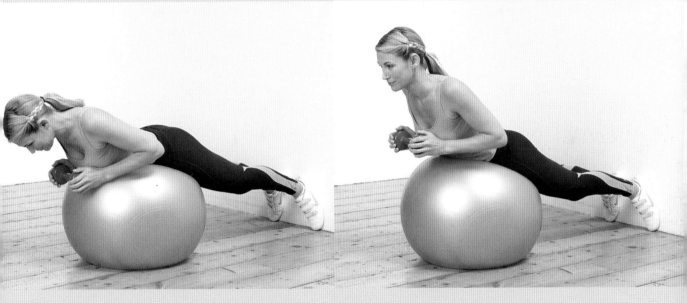

1 Lie with your stomach and hips on the ball, bracing your feet against the join of the floor and wall. Hold each end of the dumbbell with your hands against your chest. Keep your neck long and shoulders relaxed. Breathe in to prepare.

2 Breathe out, pull your navel towards your spine, and contract your buttock and back muscles as you raise your upper body. Your shoulders, hips and knees should form a line. Hold for 1 second, then breathe in and slowly lower to the start position.

deep ab-activator

Learning how to connect and strengthen your deep-seated abdominal muscles (transversus abdominis) and work your pelvic floor (pubococcygeus) will help to firm and flatten your stomach and provide support for the lower spine. This movement also stabilizes the pelvis as you move your legs. Creating a stronger, more resistant core is essential in order to progress to the full weights programme. This exercise really activates your natural 'corset' muscles.

Remember Maintain neutral spine alignment, checking that your stomach muscles stay firmly connected beneath your hands and that you avoid arching your back.

1 Lie on your back with your knees bent, and your feet flat on the mat and hip-width apart. Place your fingertips on your lower abdomen – this will ensure your stomach does not 'pop up'. Breathing normally, lift your pelvic floor and pull your navel towards your spine. Simultaneously float one leg up, so that the knee is over your hip with your leg bent at 90 degrees.

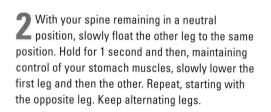

2 With your spine remaining in a neutral position, slowly float the other leg to the same position. Hold for 1 second and then, maintaining control of your stomach muscles, slowly lower the first leg and then the other. Repeat, starting with the opposite leg. Keep alternating legs.

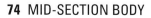

variation

As you become stronger, you will find it easier to maintain your neutral spine position for longer. The following exercise is an extension of the Deep Ab-Activator where you will continue to work the transversus. This variation provides the added challenge of working your core with both legs lifted, making your deep stomach muscles work even harder.

Remember Do not allow your back to change position throughout the movement.

1 Assume the same start position as for the Deep Ab-Activator (see step 1 opposite) but with both legs lifted and your knees over your hips, with your lower legs bent at 90 degrees. Breathe normally and pull your navel firmly towards your spine throughout.

2 Slowly lower your left foot to just off the mat, lift it back up and then repeat with your right leg.

ab-curl

EQUIPMENT mat **REPS** 12–15 **SETS** 1–3

The Ab-Curl works the abdominal muscles (rectus abdominis) that run down the centre of the abdomen from your breastbone to your pubic bone. These muscles flex your torso and are responsible for stabilizing your pelvis when walking. Strengthening them helps to give essential support to the lumbar spine. This exercise is simple but very effective.

Remember Keep your movements slow and controlled to ensure great results.

1 Lie on your back with your knees bent, and your feet flat on the mat and hip-width apart. Place your fingertips behind your ears on either side of your head. Keep your elbows open and make sure you avoid pulling on your head. Breathe in to prepare.

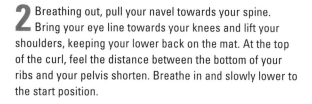

2 Breathing out, pull your navel towards your spine. Bring your eye line towards your knees and lift your shoulders, keeping your lower back on the mat. At the top of the curl, feel the distance between the bottom of your ribs and your pelvis shorten. Breathe in and slowly lower to the start position.

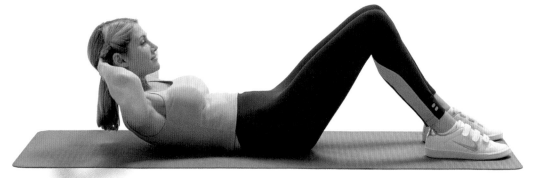

ball curl

EQUIPMENT mat, medicine ball **REPS** 12–15 **SET** 1

Another good workout for the abdominal muscles (rectus abdominis), performing the Ab-Curl with a medicine ball helps to challenge the abdominal muscles because they are working against an extra resistance. Using the medicine ball provides a refreshing alternative to the classic curl-up and can help to enhance the benefits of this movement. Use a 2 kg (4½ lb) ball to begin with.

Remember Keep a gap the size of an orange between your chin and your chest to avoid straining or tensing your neck as you curl up.

1 Lie on your back with your knees bent, and your feet flat on the mat and hip-width apart. Hold the medicine ball level with your chest, hands on either side of the ball with your elbows slightly flared away from your body. Pull your navel towards your spine throughout. Breathe in to prepare.

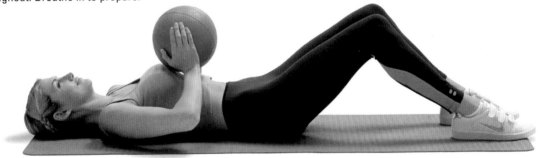

2 Breathe out and, moving your eye line towards your knees, slowly curl your shoulders and upper back forward. Keep your neck muscles relaxed. Breathe in and slowly lower to the start position.

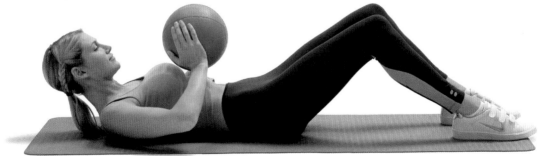

walkout

EQUIPMENT stability ball   **REPS** 5   **SET** 1

This sequence, using your abdominal muscles (rectus abdominis) and buttocks (gluteals), prepares you for the exercises where you start by lying on your back on the stability ball. Spending a few minutes learning how to get into the correct position (and off again safely!) will help you to feel more confident. You will perform each exercise with better technique and with more stability in your torso and pelvis.

Remember When returning to upright, tuck in your chin slightly, use your stomach muscles and push your back into the ball.

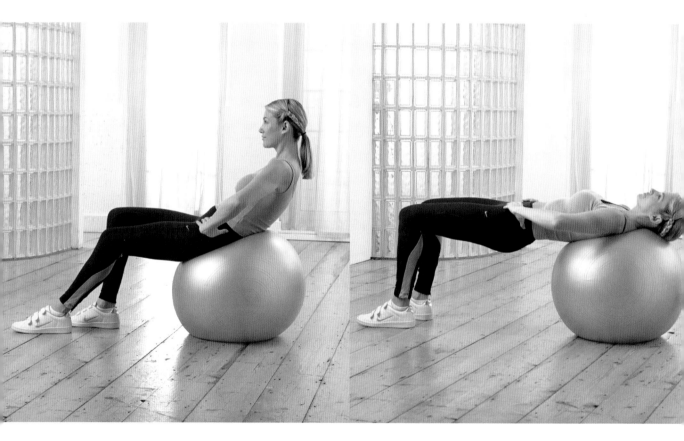

1 Sit with good posture on the ball. Hold the sides of the ball if you feel more comfortable, otherwise rest your hands on your hips. Pull your navel in towards your spine and breathe normally throughout as you slowly walk your feet away from the ball, scooping your stomach inwards.

2 Keep walking out slowly until your shoulders, neck and head rest comfortably on the ball. To return to the start position, reverse the movement, walking your feet in towards the ball as your body curves forward.

abs-olutely fabulous

EQUIPMENT stability ball   **REPS** 12–15   **SETS** 1–3

This fantastic exercise works the entire abdominal area (rectus and transversus abdominis), the buttocks (gluteals) and many of the leg muscles. The stability ball supports the hollow of your lower back, allowing your abdominals to work through a larger range of motion than is possible in floor-based abdominal work.

Remember Lift up only as far as is comfortable, keeping your movements slow and controlled.

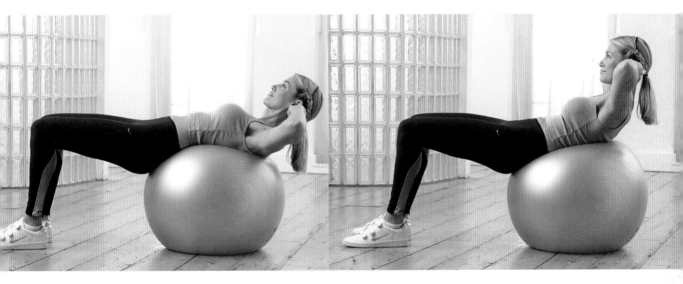

1 Sit on the ball and walk your feet out until your mid- and lower back are supported by the ball, with your knees bent and over your heels. Place your hands on either side of your head, keeping your elbows wide. Imagine holding an orange under your chin. Pull your navel towards your spine throughout. Breathe in to prepare.

2 Breathe out, lifting up your shoulders and keeping your lower back pressed firmly into the ball. Hold for 1 second, then breathe in and slowly lower to the start position.

bridge

EQUIPMENT mat   **REP** 1

This 'off the knees' modified version of the full bridge is a static exercise, which helps to strengthen the abdominal muscles (rectus abdominis), internal and external obliques, and the muscles that run the length of the spine (spinal extensors). The muscles holding the shoulder blades against the ribcage (serratus anterior) work hard to keep the shoulder blades stabilized. This is an excellent exercise to perfect good posture, helping to strengthen all your core muscles.

Remember Do not lift up your buttocks or allow your back to sag.

1 Lie face down on the mat. Begin propped up on your elbows, keeping them directly under your shoulders with your palms clasped together. Keep your eye line towards the mat. Breathe normally and pull your navel towards your spine throughout. Lift your stomach away from the mat.

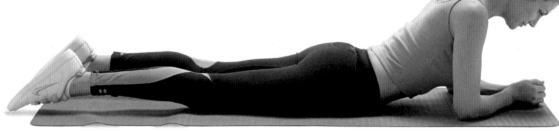

2 Raise your hips off the mat so that you are balancing on your knees. Maintain a straight line from shoulders to knees. Hold this position for 10–30 seconds, keeping your abdominal and buttock muscles firm. Lower with control.

variation

This is the full Bridge exercise, performed off the toes. It should be tried only by experienced exercisers or when you can hold the modified version easily, because it requires more strength.

Remember Do not lift up your buttocks or allow your back to sag.

1 Assume the same start position as for the modified Bridge (see step 1 opposite), with your elbows bent directly under your shoulders and palms clasped together. Tuck under your toes. Keep your eye line towards the mat. Breathe normally throughout. Pull your navel towards your spine and lift your stomach away from the mat.

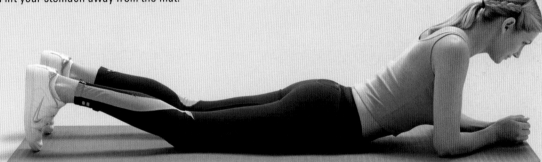

2 Keeping your shoulder blades down, raise yourself up onto your toes and elbows. Maintain a straight line from shoulders to ankles. Hold this position for 10–30 seconds, keeping your abdominal and buttock muscles firm. Lower with control.

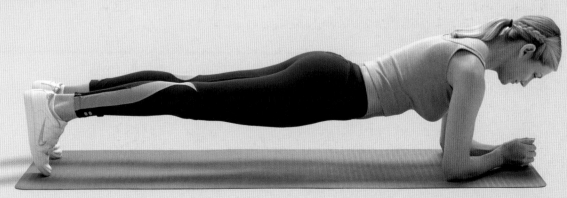

wheelbarrow

EQUIPMENT mat, stability ball **REPS** 5 **SET** 1

This is a good preparation exercise that provides the sound technique for exercises such as Half Press-ups (see page 44) and Knees-up (see page 83). Wheelbarrow improves the strength and power in the whole of your upper body, particularly your shoulder stabilizers. Your deep-seated abdominal muscles (transversus abdominis) and mid-back area will also be challenged, enhancing your overall core stability.

Remember Keep your head and neck aligned with your spine.

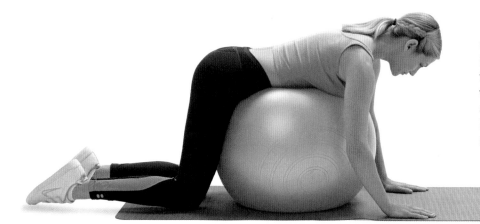

1 Kneel with the ball in front of your thighs. Breathing normally throughout, place your hands on the ball and lean forward over it, until your hands touch the floor and the ball supports your body weight. Feel how pushing into your hands supports your weight.

2 Pull your navel towards your spine to help support your hips and lower back. Push out over the ball, walking your hands out until the ball is underneath your thighs. To make it more challenging, walk out until the ball is underneath your shins. Hold for 1 second, then walk you hands back in towards the ball.

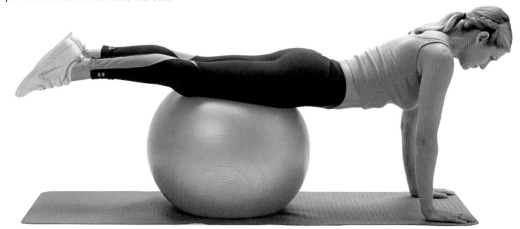

knees-up

EQUIPMENT mat, stability ball **REPS** 12–15 **SETS** 1–3

This dynamic exercise is a great way to strengthen your abdominal muscles (rectus abdominis), adding variety to your workout. The arms and lower body also work hard, with the movement of your legs forcing your abdominal muscles into action. It can be adapted to suit all levels.

Remember Keep your hips higher than your shoulders when drawing your knees in.

1 Start from the Wheelbarrow position with the ball under your shins (see opposite). Keep your shoulder blades down, pull your navel towards your spine and breathe normally throughout. Maintain a straight back and firm body and pull your toes towards the ball to hold it securely.

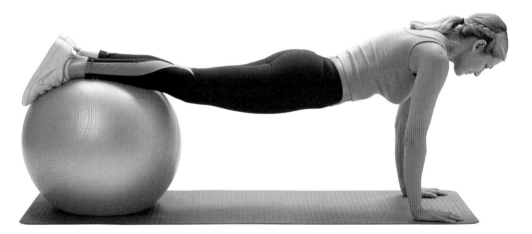

2 Keeping your eye line towards the floor, bend your knees, drawing them in towards your chest, and let the ball roll forward under your body. Hold for 1 second, then return to the start position.

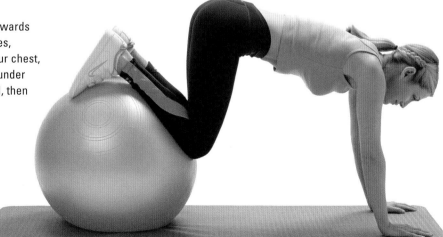

reverse curl

EQUIPMENT mat **REPS** 12–15 **SETS** 1–3

This stomach exercise targets the muscles of the lower abdomen (rectus abdominis) where the most stubborn of 'spare tyres' resides. When used as part of a balanced workout it helps to tighten, firm and improve the overall appearance of your stomach. The head and shoulders remain relaxed throughout, so the exercise is particularly good for those who tend to hold tension in the neck muscles.

Remember Try not to cheat by swinging your legs.

1 Lie on your back, bend your elbows and place your hands behind your head. Raise your legs towards the ceiling with your knees slightly bent, keeping your head and shoulders relaxed on the mat throughout. Breathe in to prepare.

2 Breathe out, contracting your lower abdominals as you pull your navel firmly towards your spine and bring your pelvis towards your ribcage. Keep the movement smooth and controlled. Breathe in and lower your hips to the mat.

torso twists

EQUIPMENT mat, foam ball   **REPS** 12–15   **SETS** 1–3

With the focus on trimming the waist muscles (internal and external obliques), this basic exercise adds shape and curves to your torso. The twisting movement works on the sides of the torso and trains the muscles that run from the ribs to the hips. Used as part of your core workout, Torso Twists produce a narrower, more defined waistline. Hold a soft ball between your knees.

Remember Squeezing the ball between your knees as you curl up activates your inner thigh muscles (adductors).

1 Lie on your back with your knees bent, and your feet flat on the mat and hip-width apart. Place your left hand to the side of your head and your right hand palm down beside your body. Breathe in to prepare, taking your eye line towards your knees.

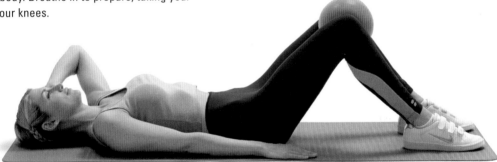

2 Breathing out, pull your navel towards your spine and curl your head and shoulders off the mat. Rotate your body, reaching through your left hand and fingertips towards your right knee. Breathe in and uncurl slowly down to the start position. Perform the required number of reps and then repeat on the opposite side.

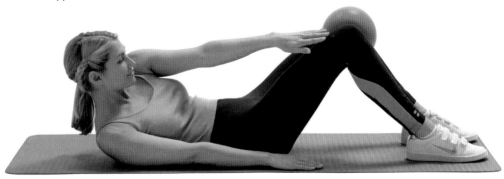

dumbbell side bends

EQUIPMENT dumbbells **REPS** 12–16 **SETS** 1–3

This is a very simple and effective exercise that targets the muscles of your waist (internal and external obliques), the abdominal muscles (rectus abdominis) and the lower back stabilizing muscles (quadratus lumborum and psoas). The muscles of the waist respond to training in various planes of movement. Dumbbell Side Bends can be practised anywhere, even without weights, to improve your curves and tighten the area overhanging the waistline of your jeans. Select suitable weights.

Remember Imagine a sheet of glass directly in front of and behind you, and you are sandwiched in between!

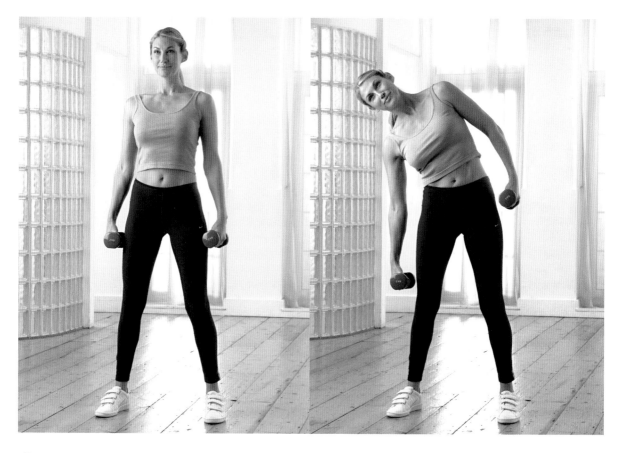

1 Stand with your feet one-and-a-half times hip-width apart and your knees soft. Hold a dumbbell in each hand with your arms by your sides and palms facing in. Breathe normally throughout, keeping your movements smooth and controlled. Keep your eye line straight ahead, and pull the top of your head towards the ceiling.

2 Pulling your navel towards your spine, drop slowly to one side. Hold your stomach firmly and feel the contraction down your sides. Avoid leaning forward or back. Maintaining control, return to the start position. Repeat on the opposite side. Keep alternating sides.

waist whittler

EQUIPMENT stability ball **REPS** 12–15 **SETS** 1–3

Whittling the muscles of the waist (internal and external obliques) and engaging your core – abdominal and back muscles – make this a challenging exercise, which calls on balance and control throughout the movement. Practised as part of a balanced workout, your waist will be trimmer and your posture will improve.

Remember Keep your head and neck aligned with your spine.

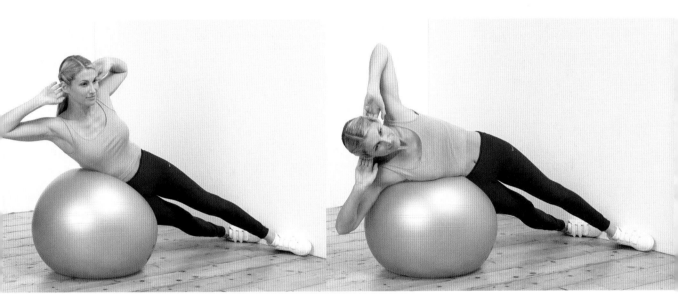

1 Brace your feet in a stride position against a step or where the floor joins the wall. Position the ball under the side of your body at hip level, with your top foot in front of your bottom foot and knees slightly bent. Pull your navel towards your spine and place your fingertips behind your head or on your temples. Keep your elbows wide and squeeze your shoulder blades together.

2 Breathe in and slowly arch your body sideways over the ball. Keep your abdominals firm and your eye line straight ahead. Breathe out as you slowly raise back up to the start position. Perform the required number of reps and then repeat on the opposite side.

suspension bridge

EQUIPMENT mat **REP** 1

The Suspension Bridge is a variation of the Bridge (see pages 80 and 81) that works more intensely on the waist muscles (internal and external obliques) as well as the abdominals. Strengthening your core, it will also help to eliminate those annoying 'love handles'. This version is suitable for more experienced exercisers.

Remember To add a dynamic challenge, don't hold the lift, but lower and lift up again immediately, gradually working up to a series of 10 reps on each side.

1 Lie on your side with your elbow under your shoulder. Your knees and hips are stacked, with one foot on top of the other. Bring your top arm under your waist. Breathe out, pulling your navel towards your spine, and contract your stomach and waist muscles strongly.

2 Now push up on your elbow, lifting your hips off the mat. Breathing normally, hold this position for 10–30 seconds. Keep lifting up the side of your waist closest to the mat, using the hand against your waist to feel the obliques working hard. Lower with control. Repeat on the opposite side.

variation

This is a modified version of the Suspension Bridge that allows you to practise this excellent exercise starting in a less intense holding position off the knees. It is a good introduction for beginners or those new to this type of static stabilization exercise.

Remember To add a dynamic challenge, don't hold the lift, but lower and lift up again immediately, gradually working up to a series of 10 reps on each side.

1 Lie on your side with your elbow under your shoulder. Your knees and hips are stacked, with your lower leg bent at 90 degrees to the knee. Bring your top arm under your waist. Breathe in to prepare and pull your navel towards your spine.

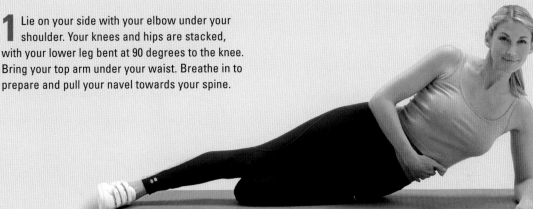

2 Breathing out, contract your stomach and waist muscles strongly, and raise your body weight up so that your lower leg and elbow support you. Breathing normally, pull up the waist muscles on the side closest to the mat and feel them tightening against your hand. Hold for 10–30 seconds. Lower with control. Repeat on the opposite side.

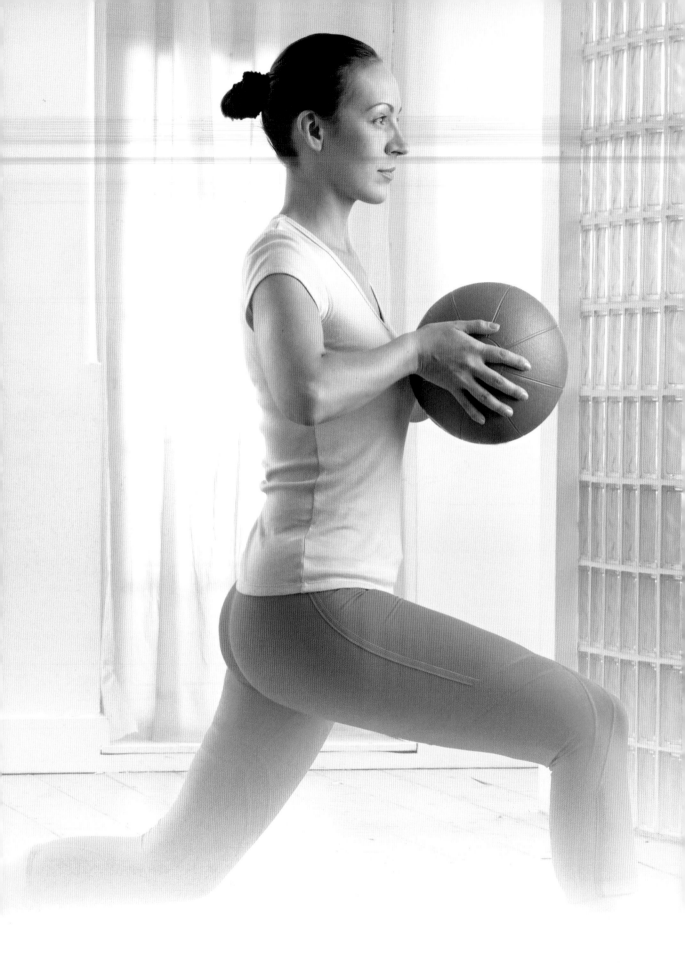

THE LOWER BODY

legs and buttocks

The muscles of your legs and buttocks need to be strong and toned to help maintain firmness and minimize the appearance of the dreaded cellulite! Resistance training is therefore essential to help establish and maintain a high ratio of muscle mass to body fat. Lean muscle is metabolically active, fat is not: the more lean muscle mass you gain, the more effectively you will burn up excess fat.

Performing exercises that build strong leg and buttock muscles will also help to prevent premature ageing and the subsequent loss of independence caused by inactivity.

Working the legs

The leg exercises in this section provide a varied workout, many targeting the stabilizing muscles that help you to balance and engage your core and buttock muscles. Use of the stability ball further enhances the training effect, providing suitable variations for all abilities.

Some of the exercises, such as the Wall Crawl, Scorpion and Ballet Buttocks, work on shaping and defining your buttocks for a firm, rounded appearance. Performed regularly, you will see lifted cheeks in no time! A variety of lunges and squats, ranging from easy to more advanced variations, combine effective sculpting and firming benefits for all areas of the thighs and buttocks. The outer thighs achieve amazing toning effects from exercises such as the Abductor Raise, and the use of ankle weights provides more resistance for optimum results.

Banish cellulite

Combined with the leg and buttock exercises, you can tackle any cellulite issues with a three-pronged approach:

- Ensure you enjoy a healthy diet and maintain adequate hydration.
- Weight train to gain and tone lean muscle, and team this with regular cardiovascular workouts to burn calories.
- Improve your circulation and any dimpled-skin appearance by dry-brushing your skin regularly in upward strokes before you shower.

You'll soon have a honed, toned physique to be proud of!

Legs and buttocks

squats

EQUIPMENT dumbbells   **REPS** 12–15   **SETS** 1–3

Working the muscles at the fronts and backs of the thighs (quadriceps and hamstrings) and buttocks (gluteals), Squats are well known for producing beautifully defined legs and firm buttocks. Squats also engage many other muscles in your body to help you achieve good technique. Select suitable weights.

Remember Do not bend your thighs below the horizontal as this will compromise back and knee safety.

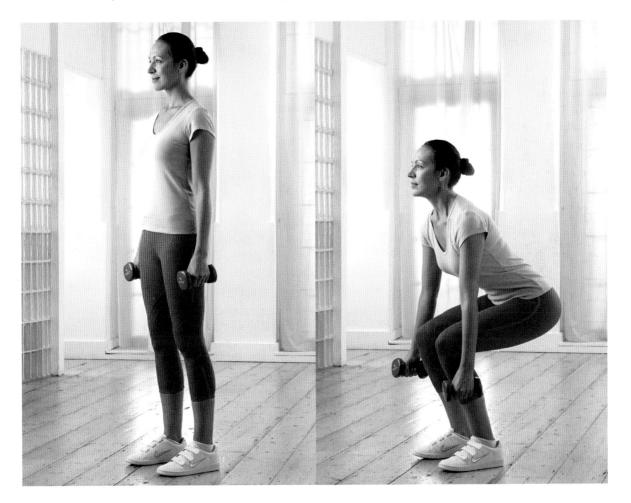

1 Stand with your feet hip-width apart and knees soft. Hold a dumbbell in each hand with your arms by your sides, palms facing in. Keep your head level and eye line straight ahead at all times. Maintain good posture and pull your navel towards your spine throughout.

2 Breathing in, bend your knees to 90 degrees and imagine you are going to perch your bottom on the edge of a chair. Keep your back straight and lean your body forward slightly. When your thighs reach horizontal (or just above), breathe out and, squeezing your buttocks, return to the start position.

raised leg squats

EQUIPMENT medicine ball **REPS** 12–15 **SETS** 1–3

Performed using the weight of a medicine ball to increase intensity, Raised Leg Squats are suitable for more experienced exercisers. They work the fronts and backs of the thighs (quadriceps and hamstrings) and buttocks (gluteals), while your inner and outer thigh muscles are also called on to stabilize you, making this a truly challenging variation. Select a 2 kg (4½ lb) medicine ball, or perform without a weight with your arms held across your chest.

Remember Ensure your supporting knee aims out over your toes as you bend. Avoid this exercise if you have knee problems.

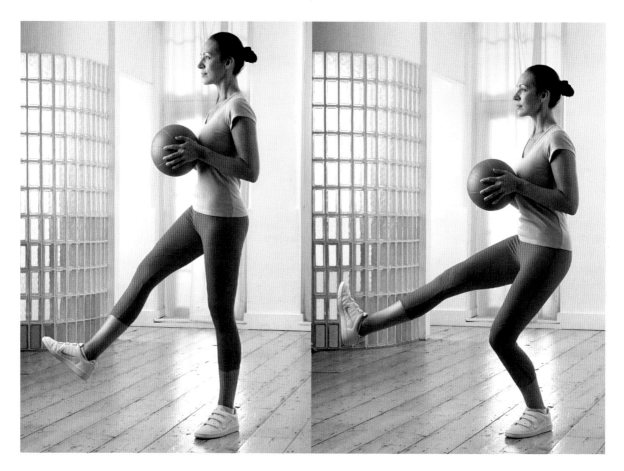

1 Stand with your feet hip-width apart and knees soft. Maintain good posture and pull your navel towards your spine throughout. Holding the ball against your chest, extend and lift one leg in front of you approximately 12–15 cm (5–6 in) off the floor. Keep your head level, eye line straight ahead and back straight.

2 Breathe in and bend your supporting knee, making sure it bends out over your toes. Bending into only a half squat, maintain stability and control throughout. Breathe out and return to the start position. Perform the required number of reps and then repeat on the opposite side.

wall crawl

EQUIPMENT stability ball, plus dumbbells for variation   **REPS** 12–15   **SETS** 1–3

Wall Crawl uses the stability ball to roll up and down the wall as you squat. It works the fronts and backs of the thighs (quadriceps and hamstrings) and the buttocks (gluteals). Practise this before you try performing any weighted squats exercises, as the return movement places less workload on your knees. The ball supports your back, making it more suitable for beginners and mature exercisers.

Remember To increase intensity, hold a dumbbell in each hand with hands beside your thighs.

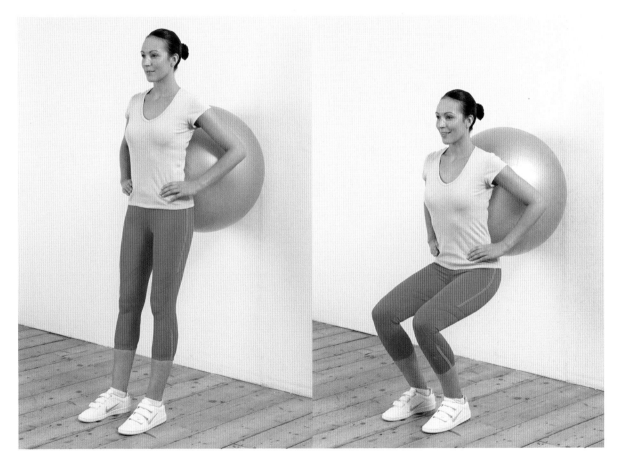

1 Place the ball against the wall between your mid- and lower- back. Keep your back straight with your hands on your hips. Walk your feet forward and, leaning your weight into the ball, position them shoulder-width apart. Keep your knees soft and in line with your ankles. Pull your navel towards your spine throughout.

2 Breathing in, slowly roll your body down until your thighs are parallel with the floor and your knees are over your ankles. Only bend as far as is comfortable. Breathing out, squeeze your buttocks and slowly roll back up to the start position.

pliés

EQUIPMENT dumbbell **REPS** 12–15 **SETS** 1–3

Pliés are originally from the ballet class and work the same muscles – fronts and backs of the thighs (quadriceps and hamstrings) and buttocks (gluteals) – as all the squat exercises (see pages 93–95), but with more emphasis on the inner thigh. The wider starting position adopted for this movement is the key to its effectiveness. Concentrate on really pushing into your heels and contracting your buttocks and inner thighs as you straighten up from the plié. Select one heavier weight.

Remember Do not allow your knees to roll in. Focus on good technique throughout.

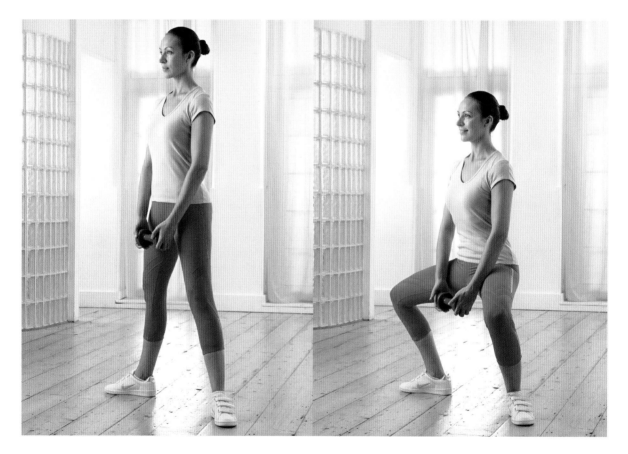

1 Hold each end of the dumbbell with your arms in front of your body. Stand with your feet one-and-a-half times shoulder-width apart, turning out your legs and feet from your hips. Keep your knees soft. Pull your navel towards your spine and keep your body upright throughout.

2 Breathe in and slowly bend your knees until your thighs are parallel to the floor (and no lower). As you bend your knees, your ankles must stay in line with them, and your knees must point out over your toes. Hold for 1 second, then breathe out and contract your inner thighs and buttocks as you push through your heels to return to the start position.

static lunge

EQUIPMENT dumbbells   **REPS** 12–15   **SETS** 1–3

Lunges are a favourite exercise for many women as they tone and define the fronts and backs of the thighs (quadriceps and hamstrings) while firming and tightening the buttocks (gluteals) and inner thighs (adductors). This static version is perfect to begin with. If you find balancing with dumbbells difficult, hold the back of a chair with one hand while performing this movement until you are confident without a support. Select suitable weights.

Remember When you bend your knees, make sure your back knee goes no deeper than 90 degrees.

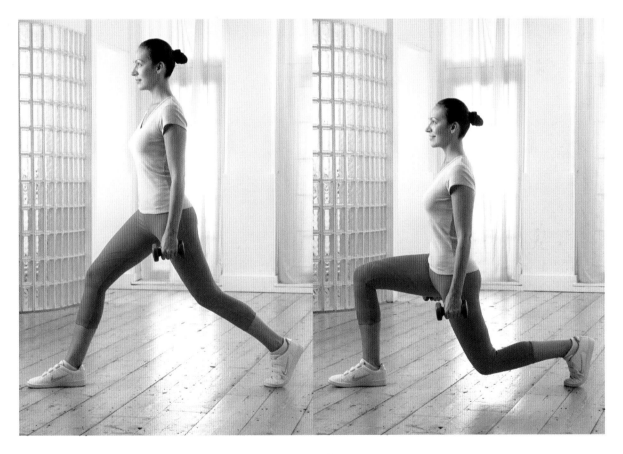

1 Stand with your feet hip-width apart and knees soft. Hold a dumbbell in each hand with your arms by your sides, palms facing in. Take a large stride forward, keeping your head level and eye line straight ahead. Pull your navel towards your spine and keep your torso upright throughout, with your back heel lifted. This is the start position.

2 Breathe in and bend both knees, keeping your weight on the heel of the front foot to engage your buttocks. Ensure your front knee does not jut out over your toes. Squeeze your buttocks, breathe out and push down into your front heel as you return to the start position. Perform the required number of reps and then repeat on the opposite side.

travelling lunges

EQUIPMENT dumbbells, plus medicine ball for variation   **REPS** 12–15   **SETS** 1–3

Increasing the intensity of the lunge by incorporating movement makes Travelling Lunges the supreme sculpting exercise for the fronts and backs of your thighs (quadriceps and hamstrings) and buttocks (gluteals). Using weights compels you to focus on maintaining good posture, balance and co-ordination. Keep this movement smooth and controlled to ensure best results. Select suitable weights.

Remember If you feel unsteady initially, practise this exercise without the dumbbells until you are more confident.

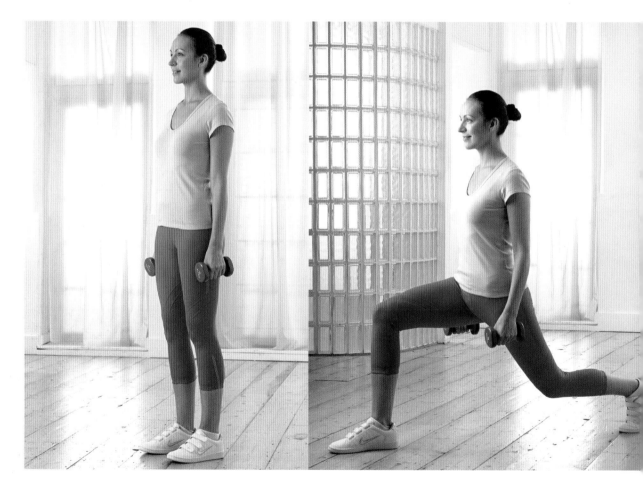

1 Stand with your feet hip-width apart and knees soft. Hold a dumbbell in each hand with your arms by your sides, palms facing in. Pull your navel towards your spine throughout. Maintain a breadth across your chest and keep your shoulder blades anchored as you move.

2 Breathe in and take a large stride forward, bending at the knee and making sure your front knee does not go past your toes. Your back knee should be no lower than 5 cm (2 in) from the floor. Keep your body still, breathe out and press down into your front heel to return to the start position. Perform 12–15 reps, then repeat on the opposite side.

variation

This advanced variation is a challenging alternative for experienced exercisers as it activates the entire body. It particularly works your thighs (quadriceps and hamstrings), buttocks (gluteals) and calves (gastrocnemius), as well as your stabilizing core muscles. Select a 2 kg (4½ lb) medicine ball.

Remember On the return movement, concentrate on pressing into your front foot.

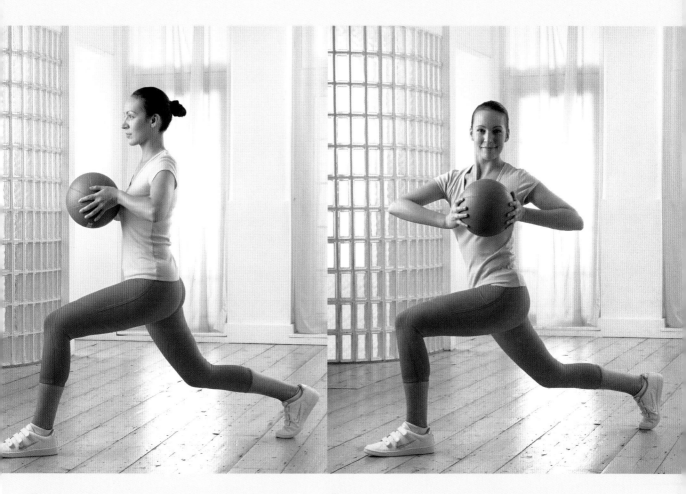

1 Hold the ball at chest level, shoulder blades anchored, feet hip-width apart, knees soft. Look straight ahead. Pulling your navel towards your spine, breathe in and take a large stride forward with your left leg into a lunge. Your front thigh should be parallel to the floor with your back knee bent at 90 degrees. Your body weight should be on your front heel.

2 Maintain this position and, holding your buttocks and abdominals firm, breathe out and rotate your upper body and the ball to the left. Breathe in as you return to the centre and, breathing out and pushing into your front heel, squeeze your buttocks and return to the start position. Repeat on the right side. Keep alternating sides.

front leg extension

EQUIPMENT chair, ankle weights, plus stability ball for variation   **REPS** 12–15   **SETS** 1–3

Strong muscles at the fronts of your thighs (quadriceps) are vital, as weakness in this area may lead to knee problems. This movement strengthens and shapes these muscles, promoting good alignment and making your knee joints more stable during everyday activities. It will also give you the confidence to wear clothes that reveal your knees! You will need 1 kg (2¼ lb) ankle weights and a chair.

Remember Avoid arching your back as your leg extends, and maintain control of your stomach muscles to hold you upright.

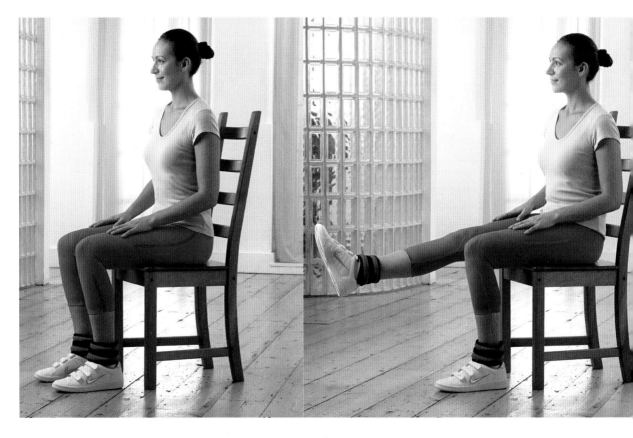

1 Sit upright on the chair with the ankle weights on, your feet flat on the floor and hip-width apart. Ensure your knees are positioned over your ankles. Hold the edge of the chair lightly, or rest your hands on top of your thighs. Breathe in to prepare.

2 Breathing out, pull your navel towards your spine and slowly raise one leg out in front of you, contracting the muscles above the kneecap and flexing your toes upwards. Hold for 1 second, then breathe in and slowly lower to the start position. Perform the required number of reps and then repeat on the opposite side.

variation

This movement is a more challenging version of the previous exercise because it is performed sitting on a stability ball. The main focus is on the balance element, requiring concentration. Working the same leg muscles, it will also cause your abdominals and back muscles to work hard to stabilize you on the ball. Select 1 kg (2¼ lb) ankle weights.

Remember Pull the top of your head up towards the ceiling. Use your abdominals and imagine your hips are headlamps – direct the beam straight ahead!

Sit upright on the ball with the ankle weights on. Position your feet flat on the floor and hip-width apart, with your knees over your ankles. Pull your navel in towards your spine throughout. Rest your hands at the sides of your hips – this will also help to keep your hips square to the front. Breathe in to prepare.

Breathing out, slowly raise one leg out in front of you, contracting the muscles above the kneecap and flexing your toes upwards. Hold for 1 second, then breathe in and return slowly to the start position. Perform the required number of reps and then repeat on the opposite side.

scorpion

This exercise gets right to the common trouble spots: the buttocks (gluteals) and backs of the thighs (hamstrings). Practise it regularly and you will soon achieve a firm, taut bottom and a sexy definition between your buttock cheeks and the back of your legs! Select 1–2 kg (2¼–4½ lb) ankle weights.

Remember Count 2 seconds as you lift, pause for 1 second and then count 2 seconds as you lower.

1 With the ankle weights on, kneel on all fours and support yourself on your elbows. Make sure your hips are over your knees and your shoulders above your elbows. Place your fists one on top of the other and rest your forehead on your top hand. Breathe in to prepare.

2 Lift your pelvic floor and pull your navel towards your spine. Breathe out and, keeping your leg bent, raise one knee to hip-height. Push up into your heel, keeping your foot flat. Breathe in and slowly lower to the start position. Perform the required number of reps and then repeat on the opposite side.

variation

For a real sting in the tail, try this standing version of the Scorpion using 1–2 kg (2¼–4½ lb) ankle weights. The advantage of this variation is that you can perform it almost anywhere, even without the ankle weights or a mat – all you need is a chair.

Remember Visualize pushing the sole of your foot against an imaginary wall close behind you. Avoid sinking your body weight into the supporting hip.

Use the back of a sturdy chair for support. Maintain good posture with your pelvic floor lifted and your navel pulled towards your spine throughout. Stand with your feet together, hold your head level and look straight ahead. Lengthen up through your spine, drawing the top of your head towards the ceiling.

Breathe in and bend one knee to 90 degrees. This is the start position. Breathe out and press the sole of your foot away from you. Breathe in and lower to the start position. Perform the required number of reps and then repeat on the opposite side.

elevator

EQUIPMENT mat, stability ball **REPS** 8–15 **SETS** 1–3

Ideal for strengthening and sculpting the buttocks (gluteals) and backs of the thighs (hamstrings), this exercise will also improve stability in your torso and increase the range of movement in your hips. The Elevator requires balance and control, and will prepare you for the more demanding variation.

Remember Keep the ball steady: don't let it wander! For a challenge, extend your arms straight up above your chest and perform this exercise.

1 Lie on your back with your heels and calves resting on the ball and your toes relaxed. Keep your legs straight without locking your knees. Place your arms by your sides, palms facing down and fingertips relaxed. Pull your navel towards your spine throughout.

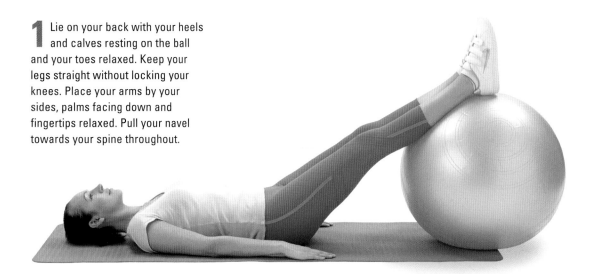

2 Tighten your buttocks, breathe in and slowly lift your hips off the mat as you push your heels down into the ball. Hold for 1 second, then breathe out and slowly lower your hips to the mat.

variation

This is an amazing exercise for the backs of your thighs (hamstrings). It uses the same movement that you will have perfected while practising the Elevator, but this variation incorporates a dragging action that really targets the hamstrings. You will also feel the effort in your calves, lower back, buttocks and core stabilizing muscles.

Remember Keep your ball movements in a straight line: imagine the ball is travelling on a railway track so it cannot drift sideways.

Assume the lifted position from the Elevator (see step 2 opposite), with your buttocks contracted and your hips lifted up. Breathe out as you push your heels into the top of the ball, pull them slowly towards you and drag the ball towards your buttocks.

Keeping your head, neck and shoulders relaxed and still, push into the ball as you breathe in and extend your legs, rolling the ball away from you. Breathe out and slowly lower your hips down to the mat.

abductor raise

EQUIPMENT mat, ankle weights, towel, plus chair for variation   **REPS** 15–20   **SETS** 1–3

Targeting the hip abductors (gluteus medius), this movement strengthens your outer buttocks. Taking the leg away from the mid-line of your body focuses the effort on the middle buttock muscles by moving the onus away from the largest buttock muscle, which often takes over. This helps to firm and shape your silhouette and give your curves definition. You will need 1 kg (2¼ kg) ankle weights and a folded towel.

Remember Look straight ahead to avoid the temptation to look down at the working leg.

1 Lie on your right side with your hips stacked. Bend your right leg slightly and extend your right arm to cushion your head. Place a folded towel between your head and right arm for good alignment. Position your left hand in front for support, relaxing your left shoulder. Pull your navel towards your spine and draw your waistline away from the mat. Breathe in to prepare.

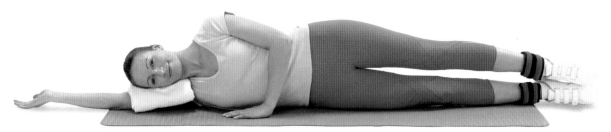

2 Breathe out, slowly lifting your left leg in line with your body with the knee facing forward. Hold for 1 second, then breathe in and lower with control to the start position. Perform the required number of reps and then repeat on the opposite side.

variation

This standing variation targets the same hip abductors as the previous exercise, but because it is performed from a standing position it also challenges your balance. Strong hip abductors are essential for any form of activity or sport involving sideways movement. You will feel the effort in both the working and supporting legs. Use 1 kg (2¼ lb) ankle weights and a chair for support.

Remember If you have a full-length mirror, use this to correct yourself. If you find using one leg continuously uncomfortable, alternate legs to begin with.

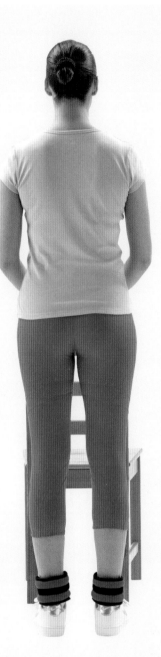

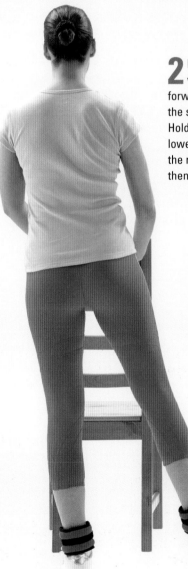

2 Keep your right leg straight with your knee and toes facing forward. Slowly raise the leg out to the side as high as is comfortable. Hold for 1 second and then slowly lower to the start position. Perform the required number of reps and then repeat on the opposite side.

1 Stand with your feet hip-width apart and knees soft. Rest your fingertips lightly on the chair back, pull your navel firmly towards your spine and look straight ahead. Your hips must remain level throughout and your posture upright to avoid leaning to one side. Breathe normally.

adductor raise

This simple exercise tones one of women's least favourite areas: the inner thighs. They are quite difficult to train effectively, but help is at hand with this movement that successfully firms and shapes these muscles (adductors). You will need 1 kg (2¼ lb) ankle weights, a folded towel and a cushion or pillow.

Remember Avoid lifting the shoulder of your supporting arm.

1 Lie on your right side with your hips stacked. Extend your right arm and rest your head on a folded towel placed between your head and arm for good alignment. Position your left arm in front for support. Bend your left leg so that the knee is in line with the hip, and rest the knee on the cushion or pillow. Pull your navel towards your spine and draw your waistline away from the mat. Breathe in to prepare.

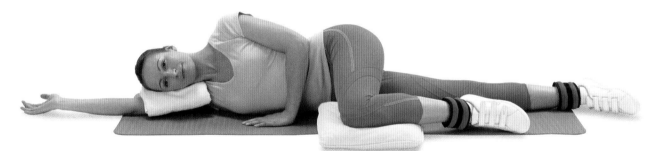

2 Breathe out as you slowly raise your right leg as high as is comfortable, contracting your inner thigh muscle. Hold for 1 second, then breathe in and slowly lower to the start position. Perform the required number of reps and then repeat on the opposite side.

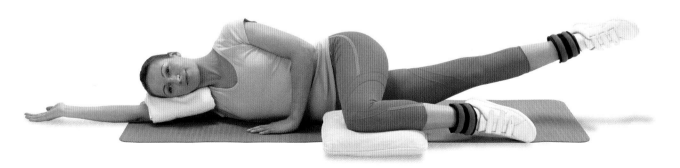

adductor refiner

EQUIPMENT chair and foam ball   **REPS** 15–20   **SETS** 1–3

This exercise can be performed just about anywhere, using a foam ball, rolled-up towel or folded pillow. It works the muscles of the inner thighs (adductors), helps to improve the overall shape and appearance of your legs, and gives you the confidence to wear your favourite clothes and swimwear. You will need a chair for support.

Remember For an extra challenge, change the tempo halfway through: after 8–10 slow releases, perform 8–10 pulses (small squeezes without releasing fully).

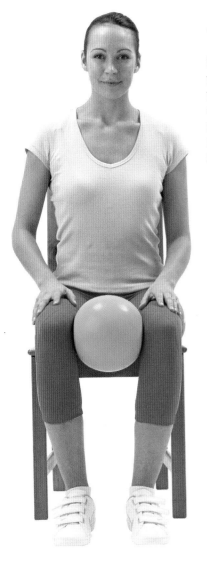

1 Sit on the edge of the chair, with your feet flat on the floor and hip-width apart and your knees over your ankles. Rest your hands on your thighs. Maintain good posture and pull your navel towards your spine throughout. Breathe normally. Place the foam ball, towel or pillow between your thighs.

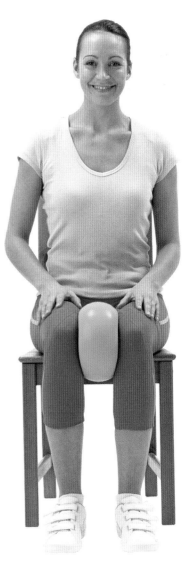

2 Squeeze your thighs firmly against the ball, keeping your body upright and feet flat. Hold for 1 second, then release very slowly and repeat immediately without resting.

debutante curtsy

EQUIPMENT dumbbells **REPS** 12–15 **SETS** 1–3

This is an effective movement suitable for experienced exercisers. The Debutante Curtsy combines working the thigh muscles (quadriceps and hamstrings), buttocks (gluteals) and your core muscles, providing an intense movement for an extra challenge in your workout. Select suitable weights.

Remember Imagine you are curtsying with a glass of water balanced on your head – don't let that water spill!

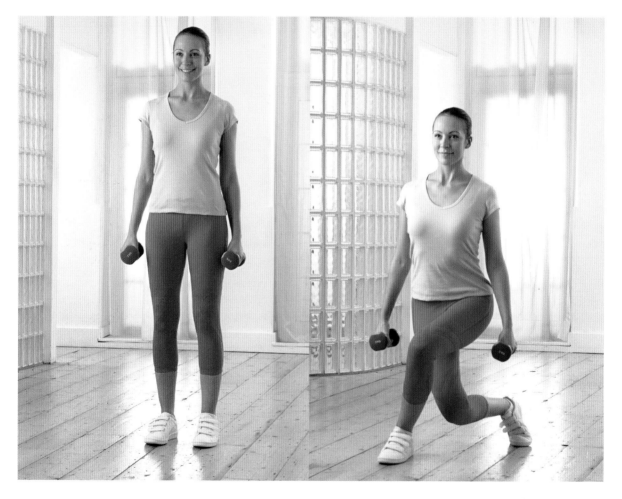

1 Stand with your feet hip-width apart and knees soft. Hold a dumbbell in each hand, with your arms by your sides and palms facing in. Maintain good posture with your back straight and pull your navel towards your spine throughout. Breathe normally.

2 Crossing your left leg in front of your right, bend both your knees into a 'curtsy', lowering your body in a straight line. Press down into your left heel and squeeze your buttocks as you return to the start position. Repeat with your right leg crossed in front of your left. Keep alternating legs.

heel hoists

EQUIPMENT chair **REPS** 12–15 **SETS** 1–3

This simple exercise concentrates on strengthening your ankle joints and creates a wonderful shape and firmness to your calf muscles (gastrocnemius and soleus). An added bonus is enhanced balance and more power for all activities, from walking to more energetic leisure and sporting activities. Use a sturdy chair or wall for support.

Remember When you find this easy, progress to standing on the edge of a stair (holding onto the banister rail for balance) and perform the same heel lifts.

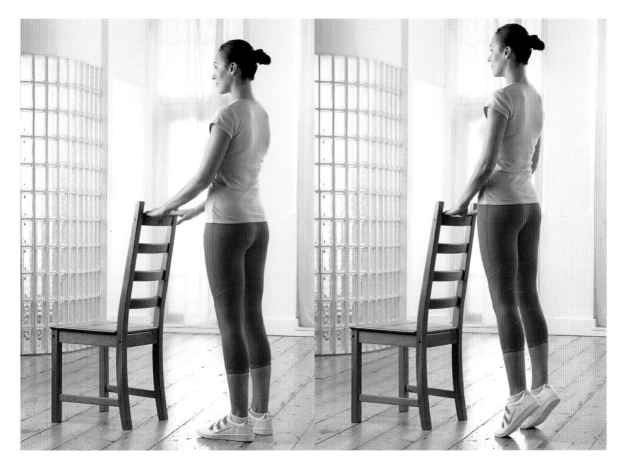

1 Place your fingertips lightly on the back of the chair or the wall to help with balance. Position your feet hip-width apart, with your knees soft. Maintain good posture and pull your navel towards your spine throughout. Keep your head level and eye line straight ahead.

2 Breathing normally, raise yourself slowly onto your tiptoes. Avoid gripping the chair back – your fingertips should just rest lightly on it. Hold for 1 second and then lower slowly to the start position.

happy feet

EQUIPMENT none   **REPS** 8–12   **SET** 1

Happy Feet is a multi-functional exercise. It not only enhances your balance and promotes flexibility in your calves, but also increases strength in the muscles that run down the fronts of your shins (tibialis anterior). Practise this regularly as a complement to Heel Hoists (see page 111) and you will quickly see an improvement in your balance and flexibility.

Remember Maintain good posture throughout and keep your navel pulled in towards your spine.

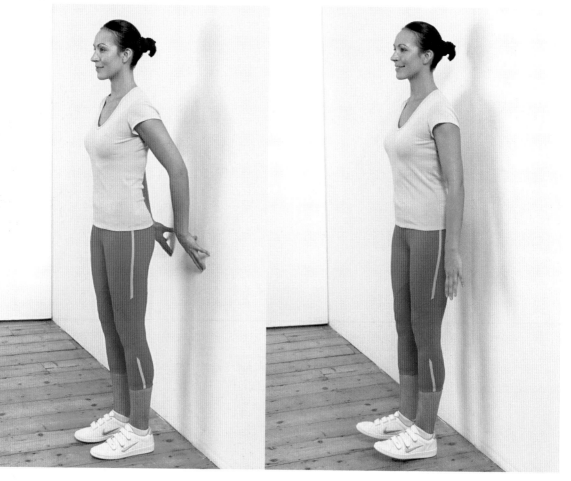

1 Stand upright with your back facing a wall and your palms resting against it. Move your heels forward by about 5 cm (2 in) so that your back does not touch the wall. Only touch the wall as a balance aid. Breathe normally.

2 Pull your navel towards your spine. Tilt your toes and the balls of your feet upwards and balance on your heels. Hold this position for 2–4 seconds, keeping your body still, then slowly lower the balls of your feet and your toes to the start position.

body raise

EQUIPMENT mat, chair **REPS** 12–15 **SETS** 1–3

The Body Raise works your buttocks (gluteals) and at the same time strengthens your back (erector spinae). Simple to perform and with no need for weights, its versatility means you can practise it as an alternative to existing buttocks exercises, or when you are away from home and may not have access to your dumbbells. You will need a sturdy bench or chair seat.

Remember Keep your upper body in alignment. Do not let your ribcage 'pop up', and maintain the straight line from knees to chest.

1 Lie on your back and place your feet on the edge of the chair seat or bench with your knees bent to 90 degrees. Your arms should rest by your sides with your palms facing down and fingertips relaxed. Pull your navel towards your spine throughout. Breathe in to prepare.

2 Breathing out, squeeze your buttocks and slowly lift your hips off the mat until there is a straight line running from your knees to your chest. Hold for 1 second, then breathe in and slowly lower to the start position.

buttock booster

EQUIPMENT mat **REPS** 10 **SET** 1

An exercise chosen with the Essential Workout (see page 118) in mind, this movement works on gaining strength in the buttocks (gluteals) without assistance from the backs of your thighs (hamstrings). Many women initially find it difficult to feel the buttock muscles working independently without other muscles taking over. This is a good basic movement for anyone new to weight training, to improve muscle awareness.

Remember As you lift your thigh, push your hipbones into the mat.

1 Lie face down with your hands resting one on top of the other, and your forehead resting on the top hand. Bend one leg so that the lower leg is at 90 degrees to the thigh. Pull your navel towards your spine throughout. Breathe normally.

2 Squeeze the buttock of the raised leg and lift the thigh a few centimetres off the mat. Hold for up to 10 seconds and then lower. Repeat on the opposite side. Keep alternating legs.

ballet buttocks

EQUIPMENT chair, ankle weights   **REPS** 8–12   **SETS** 1–2

If you want to achieve the pert buttocks you see on ballet dancers, practise this exercise! It is really a hip extension and works on strengthening the largest muscle of your buttocks (gluteus maximus) as well as the backs of thighs (hamstrings). You will achieve fantastic definition between your bottom and the back of your leg. You will also enjoy improved performance in sporting activities. You will need a chair and 1 kg (2¼ lb) ankle weights.

Remember Keep your toes pointing forward to avoid outward rotation. When you find alternating the legs easy, perform all the reps on one side, then change legs.

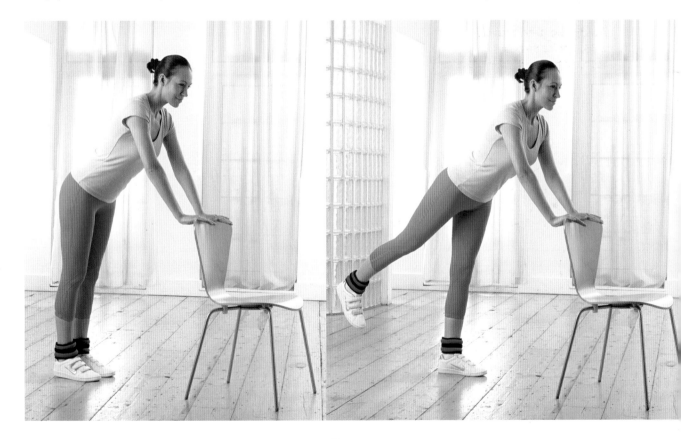

1 Stand 30–60 cm (1–2 ft) away from the chair and, leaning forward from your hips with straight legs, rest your hands lightly on the chair back. Keep your head aligned with your spine and do not tilt it up or down – fix your eye line diagonally downwards to assist. Pull your navel towards your spine throughout and breathe normally.

2 With toes pointing forward, lift your right leg straight out behind you, as high as is comfortable without forcing the lift. Do not arch your back, and keep your supporting knee soft. Hold for 1 second and then lower to the start position. Repeat with the opposite leg. Keep alternating legs.

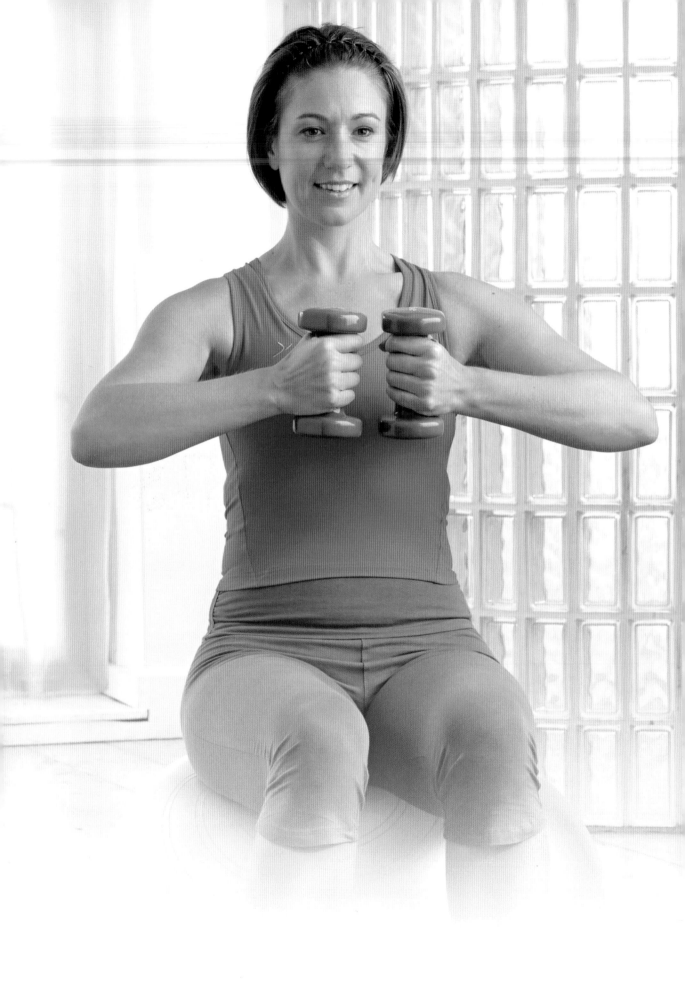

THE WORKOUTS

essential workout

This is where you begin if you have not used weights before and are out of condition. Learning essential movements is the cornerstone of a strong, resilient core and will provide you with the deep postural strength and muscular awareness that is crucial to a successful weight-training programme.

Make sure you have read the information on pages 5–21 in order to achieve the best possible results in the time you have available. Always begin with a 5-minute warm-up (see pages 24–30) and end your session with cool-down stretches. Perform the exercises in the order given. Complete 1 set of each exercise and leave at least 48 hours between workouts. Perform the Essential Workout twice a week for at least four weeks before progressing to the Easy

Workout. Make notes in your fitness diary of the exercises you have completed so that you can keep track of your progress and help you to achieve your ultimate goals.

If you miss a goal, don't panic! Revise and redefine your goals as you move on. Be disciplined. Reviewing your goals on a regular basis will help to remind you exactly what it is that you want to achieve and also reinforces the idea of where you are heading.

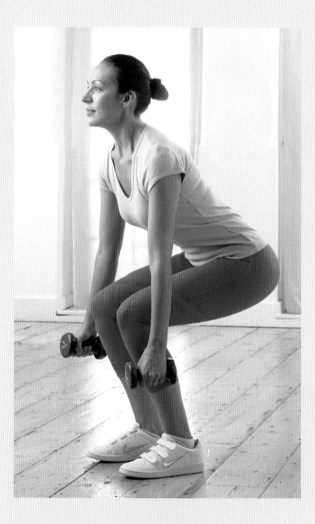

Cool-down stretches

easy workout

The Easy Workout gives you a well-structured, balanced body workout. This varied programme is the ideal starting point for those who have been practising the Essential Workout for a minimum of four weeks. If you have exercised previously, the Easy Workout is the perfect introduction to your weight training programme.

Make sure you have read the information on pages 5–21 in order to achieve the best possible results in the time you have available. Always begin with a 5-minute warm-up (see pages 24–30) and end your session with cool-down stretches. Perform the exercises in the order given. Begin with 1 set of each exercise and leave at least 48 hours between workouts. Perform the Easy Workout twice a week. As you progress, or start to find the workout easy, add

another set and increase the weight. After four to six weeks, increase the variety by replacing the Ab-Curl with the Ball Curl (see page 77), Squats with Wall Crawl (see page 95), Triceps Toner with Triceps Toner variation (see page 63) and Body Raise with Elevator (see page 104). Make notes in your fitness diary of exercises completed to keep track of your progress and help you achieve your goals.

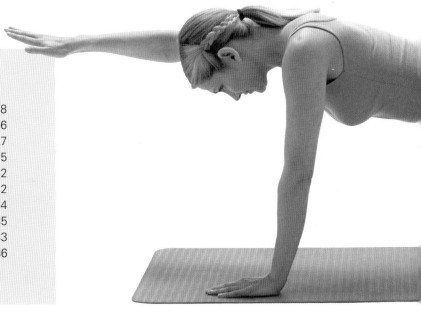

Cool-down stretches

top-to-toe workout

This workout adds challenge by using a medicine ball, dumbbells and a stability ball. To use the stability ball safely, you will need to practise the Walkout (see page 78) and the Wheelbarrow (see page 82). You will find the variety of equipment used in this top-to-toe programme makes this a stimulating and fun workout.

Make sure you have read the information on pages 5–21 in order to achieve the best possible results in the time you have available. Always begin with a 5-minute warm-up (see pages 24–30) and end your session with cool-down stretches. Perform the exercises in the order given. Begin with 1 set of each exercise and leave at least 48 hours between workouts. Perform the Top-to-toe Workout twice a week. As you progress, or start to find the workout easy, add another set and increase the weight. After four to six weeks, increase the variety by replacing Abs-olutely Fabulous with Knees-up (see page 83), Spine Extension with Spine Extension variation (see page 73), Dumbbell Pullovers with Single-Arm Row (see page 50) and Suspension Bridge with Suspension Bridge variation (see page 89). Make notes in your fitness diary of exercises completed to keep track of your progress and help you achieve your goals.

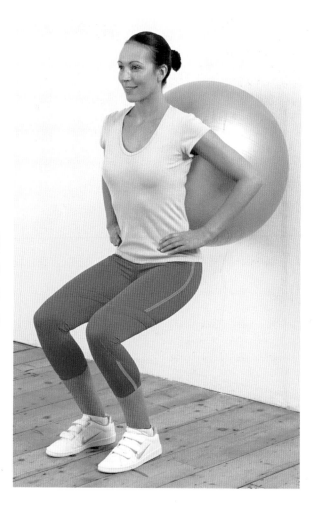

Cool-down stretches

beach body workout

To look great in your swimsuit, practise this workout for six weeks before your holiday. Combine it with regular cardiovascular work to burn excess fat, eat healthily and drink plenty of water. To use the stability ball safely, you will need to practise the Walkout (see page 78) and the Wheelbarrow (see page 82).

Make sure you have read the information on pages 5–21 in order to achieve the best possible results in the time you have available. Always begin with a 5-minute warm-up (see pages 24–30) and end your session with cool-down stretches. Perform the exercises in the order given. Begin with 1 set of each exercise and leave at least 48 hours between workouts. Perform the Beach Body Workout twice a week. As you progress, or start to find the workout

easy, add another set and increase the weight. After four to six weeks, increase the variety by replacing Travelling Lunges with Travelling Lunges variation (see page 99), Squats with Raised Leg Squats (see page 94) and Spine Extension with Spine Extension variation (see page 73). Make notes in your fitness diary of exercises completed to keep track of your progress and help you achieve your goals.

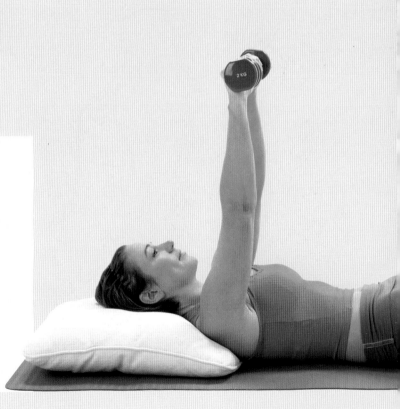

Cool-down stretches

upper body workout

A toned, defined upper body is a real confidence booster. This workout shapes the chest muscles to give the bust more lift, firms the back of the arms, melts away bra-strap fat and gives sexy shape to your shoulders! To use the stability ball safely, you will need to practise the Walkout (see page 78) and the Wheelbarrow (see page 82).

Read the information on pages 5–21 to achieve the best results in the time you have available. Begin with a 5-minute warm-up (see pages 24–30) and end your session with cool-down stretches. Perform exercises in the order given. Begin with 1 set of each exercise and leave at least 48 hours between workouts. Perform the Upper Body Workout twice a week. As you progress, or find the workout easy, add another set and increase the weight. For a short 15-minute workout, perform the

exercises marked with an asterisk*. After four to six weeks, increase variety by replacing Lateral Raise with Shoulder Shaper (see pages 54–55), Triceps Toner with Dips (see page 65), Dumbbell Side Bends with Waist Whittler (see page 87) and Hammer Curl with Biceps Beautifier (see page 59) or Hammer Curl variation (see page 61). Make notes in your fitness diary of exercises completed to keep track of your progress and help you achieve your goals.

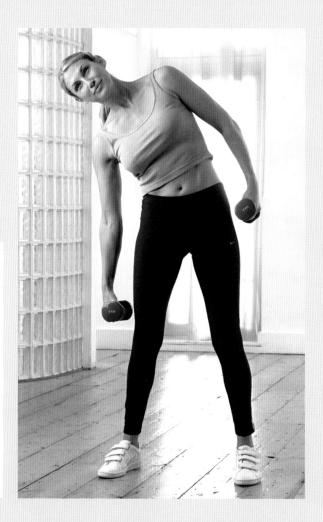

Cool-down stretches

lower body workout

To achieve firm, lissom legs and a pert derrière, you must focus on exercises that work the relevant muscles through different ranges of motion. For best results, combine this workout with regular power walking and/or cycling. To use the stability ball safely, you will need to practise the Walkout (see page 78) and the Wheelbarrow (see page 82).

Read the information on pages 5–21 in order to achieve the best results in the time you have available. Always begin with a 5-minute warm-up (see pages 24–30) and end your session with cool-down stretches. Perform the exercises in the order given. Begin with 1 set of each exercise and leave at least 48 hours between workouts. Perform the Lower Body Workout twice a week. As you progress, or start to find the workout easy, add another set and increase the weight. For a short 15-minute workout, perform the exercises marked with an asterisk*. After four to six weeks, increase the variety by replacing the Scorpion with the Scorpion variation (see page 103), Travelling Lunges with Travelling Lunges variation (see page 99) and Front Leg Extension with Front Leg Extension variation (see page 101). Make notes in your fitness diary of exercises completed to keep track of your progress and help you achieve your goals.

Travelling Lunges*	page 98
Front Leg Extension*	page 100
Ballet Buttocks*	page 115
Abductor Raise (variation)*	page 107
Adductor Refiner*	page 109
Debutante Curtsy	page 110
Elevator (variation)	page 105
Abductor Raise	page 106
Adductor Raise	page 108
Scorpion	page 102

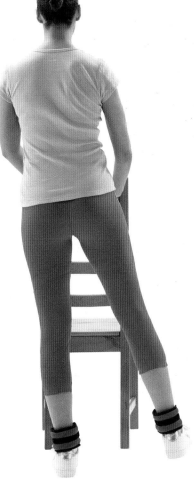

Cool-down stretches

Adductor Stretch	page 39
Abductor Stretch	page 39
Buttock Stretch	page 38
Prone Hamstring Stretch	page 38
Front of Hip Stretch	page 36
Spinal Rotation	page 35
Standing Cat Stretch	page 33
Calf Stretch	page 31
Front of Leg Stretch	page 31

back workout

Targeting deep-seated abdominal and spinal muscles and improving strength in the mid-back helps to improve posture and give a strong, resilient back. However, if you do have back problems, consult your doctor before starting this programme. To use the stability ball safely, you will need to practise the Walkout (see page 78) and the Wheelbarrow (see page 82).

Make sure you have read the information on pages 5–21 in order to achieve the best possible results in the time you have available. Always begin with a 5-minute warm-up (see pages 24–30) and end your session with cool-down stretches. Perform the exercises in the order given. Begin with 1 set of each exercise and leave at least 48 hours between workouts. Perform the Back Workout twice a week. As you progress, or start to find the workout easy,

add another set and increase the weight. Make notes in your fitness diary of exercises completed to keep track of your progress and help you to achieve your goals.

If you miss a goal, don't panic! Revise and redefine your goals as you move on. Be disciplined. Reviewing your goals on a regular basis will help to remind you exactly what it is that you want to achieve and also reinforces the idea of where you are heading.

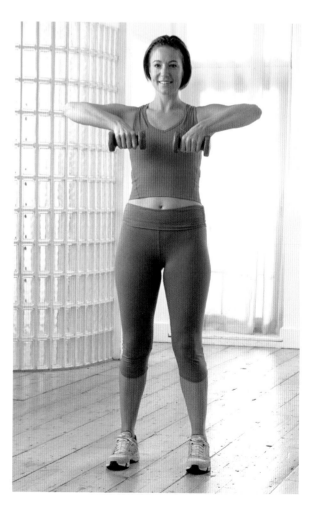

Cool-down stretches

mature woman workout

This programme offers a range of gentle exercises designed to enhance mobility, improve balance, and provide essential strength and flexibility without placing undue stress on the joints. It is suitable for mature, overweight or very unfit women. To use the stability ball safely, you will need to practise the Walkout (see page 78) and the Wheelbarrow (see page 82).

Make sure you have read the information on pages 5–21 in order to achieve the best possible results in the time you have available. Always begin with a 5-minute warm-up (see pages 24–30) and end your session with cool-down stretches. Perform the exercises in the order given. Begin with 1 set of each exercise and leave at least 48 hours between workouts. Perform the Mature Woman's Workout twice a week. As you progress, or start to find the workout easy, add another set, but always select light weights when using dumbbells. Make notes in your fitness diary of exercises completed to keep track of your progress and help you achieve your goals.

If you miss a goal, don't panic! Revise and redefine your goals as you move on. Be disciplined. Reviewing your goals on a regular basis will help to remind you exactly what it is that you want to achieve and also reinforces the idea of where you are heading.

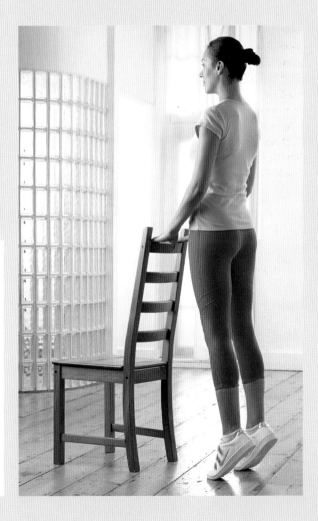

Cool-down stretches

index

acknowledgements

A big thank you goes to Michael Harrison for his help and unfaltering encouragement in the writing of this book. My appreciation goes to my clients, who continue to inspire me with their enthusiasm for my teaching methods and for the results they achieve. Thank you also to the team at Hamlyn for their friendly guidance and help, and to Mike Prior for his excellent photography. A special mention goes to my family for their infinite patience and support.

Executive Editor Jane McIntosh
Senior Editor Lisa John
Executive Art Editor Darren Southern
Designer Peter Gerrish
Picture Research Jennifer Veall
Senior Production Controller Martin Croshaw

Picture Acknowledgements
Special Photography:
© Octopus Publishing Group Limited/Mike Prior.

Other Photography:
Corbis UK Ltd/Rick Gomez 21;
Octopus Publishing Group Limited/Russell Sadur 8, 11.